ESSENTIAL MATH *and* CALCULATIONS *for* PHARMACY TECHNICIANS

CRC PRESS PHARMACY EDUCATION SERIES

Pharmacoethics: A Problem-Based Approach
David A. Gettman and Dean Arneson

Pharmaceutical Care: Insights from Community Pharmacists
William N. Tindall and Marsha K. Millonig

Essentials of Law and Ethics for Pharmacy Technicians
Kenneth M. Strandberg

Essentials of Pharmacy Law
Douglas J. Pisano

Essentials of Pathophysiology for Pharmacy
Martin M. Zdanowicz

Pharmacy: What It Is and How It Works
William N. Kelly

Pharmacokinetic Principles of Dosing Adjustments: Understanding the Basics
Ronald Schoenwald

Strauss's Federal Drug Laws and Examination Review, Fifth Edition
Steven Strauss

Pharmaceutical and Clinical Calculations, Second Edition
Mansoor Khan and Indra Reddy

Inside Pharmacy: Anatomy of a Profession
Ray Gosselin, Jack Robbins, and Joseph Cupolo

Understanding Medical Terms: A Guide for Pharmacy Practice, Second Edition
Mary Stanaszek, Walter Stanaszek, and Robert Holt

Pharmacokinetic Analysis: A Practical Approach
Peter Lee and Gordon Amidon

Guidebook for Patient Counseling
Harvey Rappaport, Tracey Hunter, Joseph Roy, and Kelly Straker

ESSENTIAL MATH *and* CALCULATIONS *for* PHARMACY TECHNICIANS

INDRA K. REDDY
MANSOOR A. KHAN

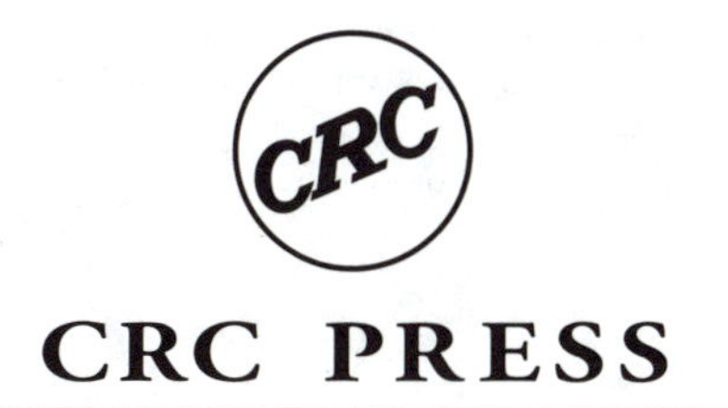

CRC PRESS

Boca Raton London New York Washington, D.C.

Library of Congress Cataloging-in-Publication Data

Reddy, Indra K.
Essential math and calculations for pharmacy technicians / Indra K. Reddy, Mansoor Khan.
p. cm. -- (CRC Press pharmacy education series)
Includes index.
ISBN 1-58716-147-8
1. Pharmaceutical arithmetic. I. Khan, Mansoor A. II. Title. III. Series.

RS57.R43 2003
615′.14′01513—dc22 2003055405

Direct all inquiries to CRC Press LLC, 2000 N.W. Corporate Blvd., Boca Raton, Florida 33431.

Visit the CRC Press Web site at www.crcpress.com

International Standard Book Number 1-58716-147-8
Library of Congress Card Number 2003055405
Printed in the United States of America 1 2 3 4 5 6 7 8 9 0
Printed on acid-free paper

Preface

The precise and accurate calculation of medication dosages is the most critical element in providing pharmaceutical care and for achieving optimal patient outcomes. It is the primary responsibility of every healthcare professional who is involved in compounding, handling, counseling and/or administering drugs to carry out medication orders efficiently and precisely.

Unfortunately, medication errors happen in pharmacies, in hospitals, or even at home or in homecare settings. Sometimes, even minor dosage calculation errors can be dangerous to the patient and may prove very costly. Ability to learn and perform the basic math are important criteria for any healthcare professional. Careful, systematic calculation and a conceptual understanding of pharmacy math are therefore essential in providing optimal medical and pharmaceutical care.

The present text is directed to the student or professional who has difficulty with basic pharmacy math. Specifically, the book is recommended for pharmacy technicians, first-year pharmacy students (as a self-study guide or for remedial math training to catch up with advanced pharmacy math), nurse practitioners and other allied health professionals, or as a reference book in pharmacies.

This book presents information in a simple and clear way, organized in a natural progression from basic principles to more complex information. The topics include Roman and Arabic numerals, fractions, decimals, ratios, proportions, percentages, systems of measurement including household conversions, interpretation of medication orders, errors and omissions, isotonicity, pH, buffers, reconstitutions, calories, intravenous flow rates, and units of biologic products. Calculations associated with liquid and solid dosage forms have been addressed separately under two separate chapter headings dealing with each type. In addition, problems associated with temperature conversions, capsule dosage forms, special considerations in pediatric dosages, and pharmacy business math have been addressed in Appendices A through D.

The book is designed in such a way that it provides math basics in a stepwise fashion, explains the fundamental concepts where needed, presents many solved examples in each chapter, and provides ample practice opportunities. The goal is to facilitate students' understanding of the material and mastery of the basic math, eventually instilling confidence in their ability to perform accurate calculations. The information presented has been thoroughly classroom tested with proven successful results. However, this book should be used exclusively as a learning tool and not as a source of information for professional practice.

The authors would like to acknowledge with thanks the participation and input of many professional colleagues, pharmacists, and professional pharmacy students who helped organize the material and who supplied examples for various topics within this text.

Indra K. Reddy
Mansoor A. Khan

Table of Contents

1 Working with Roman and Arabic Numerals

ROMAN NUMERALS

The Romans were active in trade and commerce, and from the time of learning to write they needed a way to indicate numbers. The system they developed lasted many centuries and is still in use in some areas, including pharmacy. Roman numerals are used with the apothecary's system of measurement to designate quantities on prescriptions. In the Roman system of counting, letters of the alphabet (both uppercase and lowercase) such as I or i, V or v, and X or x are used to designate numbers.

Examples:

4 = IV
12 = XII
19 = XIX
25 = XXV
49 = XLIX or IL

Rules

In the usage of Roman numerals, the following set of rules applies:

1. Roman numerals have no symbol for zero. This makes computations very difficult.
2. The numbers are written starting from the largest number on the left, and adding smaller numbers to the right. When Roman numeral(s) of lesser value follow one of a greater value, they are added.

   Examples:
   VII = 5 + 1 + 1 = 7
   XVI = 10 + 5 + 1 = 16
   CLX = 100 + 50 + 10 = 160

3. When a Roman numeral of lesser value precedes one of a greater value, it is subtracted from the greater value numeral. However, this rule only works for one small numeral before one larger numeral. For example, IX is 9 but IIX is not 8; it is not a recognized Roman numeral.

Examples:
IV = 5 – 1 = 4
IX = 10 – 1 = 9
XL = 50 – 10 = 40

4. When a Roman numeral of a lesser value is placed between two greater values, it is first subtracted from the greater numeral placed after it, and then that value is added to the other numeral(s) (i.e., subtraction rule applies first, then the addition rule).

   Examples:
   XXIX = 10 + 10 + (10 – 1) = 29
   XIV = 10 + (5 – 1) = 14

5. There is no place value in this system. For example, the number III is 3 and not 111. Also, when a Roman numeral is repeated, it doubles its value; when a Roman numeral is repeated three times, it triples its value.

   Examples:
   I = 1; II = 2; III = 3
   X = 10; XX = 20; XXX = 30

   Note. Roman numerals may not be repeated more than three times in succession. For example, 4 is written as IV but not as IIII, and 40 is written as XL but not XXXX.
6. When possible, largest value numerals are used. For example, 15 is written as XV but not as VVV.
7. Roman numerals are sometimes combined with the abbreviation for one half, ss. The abbreviation should always be at the end of a Roman numeral. Generally, Roman numerals are written in lowercase when used with ss, such as iss to indicate 1½.

Selected Roman numerals and their Arabic equivalents are shown in Table 1.1.

ARABIC NUMERALS

Arabic numerals are the most common symbols used to represent numbers. Every number can be expressed in Arabic numerals by using 10 basic symbols, alone or in combination. The basic symbols, called digits, are: 0, 1, 2, 3, 4, 5, 6, 7, 8, and 9. The position of a digit in an Arabic numeral determines its value.

Examples:
The Arabic numeral for the number two hundred and thirty-seven is the sequence of digits 237. In this numeral, the digit 2 has a value of two hundred, the digit 3 has a value of thirty, and the digit 7 has a value of seven.

TABLE 1.1
Roman and Arabic Numerals

Units		Tens		Hundreds		Thousands		Tens of Thousands		Hundreds of Thousands	
Arabic #	Roman #	Arabic #	Roman #	Arabic #	Roman #	Arabic #	Roman #	Arabic #	Roman #	Arabic #	Roman #
1	I	10	X	100	C	1000	M	10,000	$\overline{X}$	100,000	$\overline{C}$
2	II	20	XX	200	CC	2000	MM	20,000	$\overline{X}\overline{X}$	200,000	$\overline{C}\overline{C}$
3	III	30	XXX	300	CCC	3000	MMM	30,000	$\overline{X}\overline{X}\overline{X}$	300,000	$\overline{C}\overline{C}\overline{C}$
4	IV	40	XL	400	CD	4000	$M\overline{V}$	40,000	$\overline{X}\overline{L}$	400,000	$\overline{C}\overline{D}$
5	V	50	L	500	D	5000	$\overline{V}$	50,000	$\overline{L}$	500,000	$\overline{D}$
6	VI	60	LX	600	DC	6000	$\overline{V}M$	60,000	$\overline{L}\overline{X}$	600,000	$\overline{D}\overline{C}$
7	VII	70	LXX	700	DCC	7000	$\overline{V}MM$	70,000	$\overline{L}\overline{X}\overline{X}$	700,000	$\overline{D}\overline{C}\overline{C}$
8	VIII	80	LXXX	800	DCCC	8000	$\overline{V}MMM$	80,000	$\overline{L}\overline{X}\overline{X}\overline{X}$	800,000	$\overline{D}\overline{C}\overline{C}\overline{C}$
9	IX	90	XC	900	CM	9000	$M\overline{X}$	90,000	$\overline{X}\overline{C}$	900,000	$\overline{C}\overline{M}$

Note. Roman numerals can be written in big or small letters (i.e., I or i, V or v, etc). Also note that tens and hundreds of thousands are written similar to tens and hundreds, respectively, except that they have a bar on each letter.

The Arabic numeral for the number seven thousand and three is 7003. In this case, the digit 7 has a value of seven thousand, and the digit 3 has a value of three. The digit 0 (zero) fills empty positions so that the other digits have their proper values.

The numbers 0, 1, 2, 3, 4, 5, 6, 7, 8, and 9 are used throughout the world for all scientific and trade purposes. The system was developed in India in the 9th century, reaching Europe and the rest of the world through the Arab countries, where the place-value aspect of the system, with 10 as the base, developed. The use of zero and the place-values enabled the system to replace the Roman numerals then in use. All forms of computation can be carried out efficiently using the Arabic system, whereas calculations using Roman numerals are extremely cumbersome.

PRACTICE PROBLEMS

1. Express the following Arabic numerals as Roman numerals.

a. 38	h. 127	o. 155
b. 15	i. 69	p. 1782
c. 17	j. 135	q. 942
d. 91	k. 473	r. 355
e. 23	l. 864	s. 420
f. 43	m. 1223	t. 925
g. 54	n. 862	

2. Convert the following Roman numerals into Arabic numerals.

a. VIII	h. MXL	o. CDLII
b. XXV	i. XCIX	p. MCMLXVI
c. XXIII	j. XLI	q. XCVI
d. IIX	k. DCL	r. CXIV
e. XIX	l. XXVII	s. LXIV
f. MC	m. CXLIX	t. CLXXVII
g. CD	n. CCXL	

3. Perform the following operations and provide the answers in Arabic numerals.

a. VII + LXIV	f. MC – CCXL
b. XXV × CXIII	g. CD + CXLIX
c. CDL – XIX	h. MXL – XLI
d. XII + XXVII	i. MMMDCCCXL ÷ CXX
e. XIX + MCMLXVI	j. CXVII + CLXVI

4. Complete the following operations and provide the results in Roman numerals.

   a. 12 + 16
   b. 24 + 35
   c. 182 + 133 + 145
   d. 120 – 21
   e. 1589 – 39
   f. 1845 – 123
   g. 625 × 15
   h. 25 × 150
   i. 8750 ÷ 50
   j. 1904 ÷ 8

5. Interpret the quantity in each of the following:

   a. Caplets no. xxv
   b. Pills no. clxx
   c. Tablets no. mdcl
   d. Capsules no. xlv
   e. Tablets no. lxix

ANSWERS

1. Answers are presented as Roman numerals:

   a. XXXVIII
   b. XV
   c. XVII
   d. XCI
   e. XXIII
   f. XLIII
   g. LIV
   h. CXXVII
   i. LXIX
   j. CXXXV
   k. CDLXXIII
   l. DCCCLXIV
   m. MCCXXIII
   n. DCCCLXII
   o. CLV
   p. MDCCLXXXII
   q. CMXLII
   r. CCCLV
   s. CDXX
   t. CMXXV

2. Answers are presented as Arabic numerals:

   a. 8
   b. 25
   c. 23
   d. Not a recognized number
   e. 19
   f. 1100
   g. 400
   h. 1040
   i. 99
   j. 41
   k. 650
   l. 27
   m. 149
   n. 240
   o. 452
   p. 1966
   q. 96
   r. 114
   s. 64
   t. 177

3. Answers are presented in Arabic numerals:

   a. 71
   b. 2825
   c. 431
   d. 39
   e. 1985
   f. 860
   g. 549
   h. 999
   i. 32
   j. 283

4. Answers are presented as Roman numerals:

   a. XXVIII
   b. LIX
   c. CDLX
   d. XCIX
   e. MDL
   f. MDCCXXII
   g. M$\overline{X}$CCCLXXV
   h. MMMDCCL
   i. CLXXV
   j. CCXXXVIII

5. Answers are presented in Arabic numerals:

   a. 25
   b. 170
   c. 1650
   d. 45
   e. 69

2 Using Fractions and Decimals in Pharmacy Math

FRACTIONS

A *fraction* indicates a portion of a whole number. Fractions contain two numbers: the bottom number (referred to as *denominator*) and the top number (referred to as *numerator*). The denominator in the fraction is the total number of parts into which the whole is divided. The top number or numerator indicates how many of those parts are considered.

$$\frac{3}{4} = \frac{\text{numerator}}{\text{denominator}}$$

There are two types of fractions: a) *common fractions*, such as ¼ and ¾ (referred to simply as fractions) and b) *decimal fractions*, such as 0.25 or 0.75 (usually referred as decimals).

Following are some important terms in dealing with fractions:

1. Proper fractions. A *proper fraction* should always be less than 1, i.e., the numerator is smaller than the denominator:

   $$\boxed{\frac{A}{B}} \text{ where, A < B}$$

   A proper fraction such as 3/5 may be read as "3 of 5 parts" or as "3 divided by 5."

   Examples: 3/4, 5/7, 2/7

2. Improper fractions. An improper fraction has a numerator that is greater than or equal to the denominator.

   $$\boxed{\frac{A}{B}} \text{ where, A} \geq \text{B}$$

   Examples: 5/3, 19/7, 7/4

Note. If the values of both numerator and denominator are the same, the value of the fraction is equal to 1. For example, 4/4 = 1 or 5/5 = 1

3. Mixed fractions. In mixed fractions, a whole number and a proper fraction are combined. The value of the mixed fraction is always greater than 1.

$$\boxed{C\frac{A}{B}} \text{ where C is a whole number}$$

Examples: $2\frac{3}{4}$, $1\frac{5}{8}$, $1\frac{2}{3}$

Note. Improper and mixed fractions are interchangeable. This can be done according to the following formula:

$$\boxed{\frac{A}{B} = C\frac{D}{B} = \frac{(B \times C) + D}{B}}$$

where A > B (i.e., improper fraction).

Examples:

$$\frac{12}{5} = 2\frac{2}{5} = \frac{(5 \times 2) + 2}{5}$$

$$\frac{4}{3} = 1\frac{1}{3} = \frac{(1 \times 3) + 1}{3}$$

4. Complex fractions. In complex fractions, the numerator or the denominator, or both, may be a whole number, proper fraction, or mixed fraction. The value of complex fractions can be less than or greater than 1.

$$\boxed{\frac{A}{B}} \text{ where A and B are any kinds of fractions.}$$

Examples:

$$5/8 \div 1/3 = [5/8]/[1/3]$$

$$2/3 \div 7/8 = [2/3]/[7/8]$$

5. Equivalent fractions. Fractions that represent the same number are called equivalent fractions. For example, 1/2, 2/4, and 4/8 are all equivalent fractions.

$$\boxed{\frac{A}{B} = \frac{A \times C}{B \times C}}$$

$$\frac{3}{5}=\frac{3\times 2}{5\times 2}=\frac{6}{10}$$

Hence 3/5 and 6/10 are considered equivalent fractions.

To perform dosage calculations, one must be able to convert among different types of fractions and reduce them to lowest terms. One should be able to apply the basic operations of addition, subtraction, multiplication, and division. A review of these simple rules of working with fractions is provided below.

To reduce the improper fraction, divide the numerator by the denominator.

Examples:

$7/4 = 7 \div 4 = 1\frac{3}{4}$
$9/4 = 9 \div 4 = 2\frac{1}{4}$

To reduce the fraction to its *lowest terms* (which may be referred to as "simplifying the fraction"), divide numerator and denominator with the largest number that will evenly divide each term.

Examples:

$8/12 = (8 \div 4)/(12 \div 4) = 2/3$
$9/27 = (9 \div 9)/(27 \div 9) = 1/3$

Addition of Fractions

To add fractions, the following steps may be used:

1. Find a *least common denominator* (LCD) or the smallest number that divides all the denominators evenly.
2. Change each fraction so that it has that denominator but retains its original value.
3. Add the numerators.
   Note: The denominators can never be added or subtracted.
4. Reduce the resulting fraction to its lowest terms.

$$\boxed{\frac{A}{B}+\frac{C}{B}+\frac{D}{B}=\frac{A+C+D}{B}}$$

Example 1:

4. Reduce the resulting fraction to its lowest terms.

A. Adding fractions that have same denominators:

$$\frac{2}{5}+\frac{3}{5}+\frac{4}{5}=\frac{2+3+4}{5}=\frac{9}{5}=1\frac{4}{5}$$

B. Adding fractions that have different denominators:

$$\frac{1}{2}+\frac{2}{3}$$

The LCD in this case is 6 (2 × 3), which is evenly divided by each denominator. Using this LCD, the problem can be expressed as follows:

$$\frac{1\times 3}{2\times 3}+\frac{2\times 2}{3\times 2}=\frac{3}{6}+\frac{4}{6}$$

$$\frac{3+4}{6}=\frac{7}{6}=1\frac{1}{6}$$

Example 2: Find the sum of:

$$\frac{1}{6}+\frac{3}{8}$$

The LCD for 6 and 8 is 24 (24/6 = 4 and 24/8 = 3)

$$\frac{1\times 4}{6\times 4}+\frac{3\times 3}{8\times 3}=\frac{4}{24}+\frac{9}{24}$$

$$\frac{4+9}{24}=\frac{13}{24}$$

Example 3: Find the sum of:

$$\frac{3}{4}+\frac{1}{2}$$

The LCD for 4 and 2 = 4 (4/4 = 1 and 4/2 = 2)

$$\frac{3\times 1}{4\times 1}+\frac{1\times 2}{2\times 2}=\frac{3}{4}+\frac{2}{4}$$

$$\frac{3+2}{4}=\frac{5}{4}$$

Note. This can presented as a mixed fraction as follows:

$$\frac{5}{4}=1\frac{1}{4}$$

Some numbers are expressed as mixed numbers (a whole number and a fraction). To change mixed numbers to improper fractions, multiply the whole number by the denominator of the fraction and then add the numerator.

$$A\frac{B}{C} = \frac{(A \times C) + B}{C}$$

Example 1: Find the sum of:

$$3\frac{1}{4} + 5\frac{1}{16}$$

The first fraction:

$$3\frac{1}{4} = \frac{(3 \times 4) + 1}{4} = \frac{12 + 1}{4} = \frac{13}{4}$$

The second fraction:

$$5\frac{1}{16} = \frac{(5 \times 16) + 1}{16} = \frac{80 + 1}{16} = \frac{81}{16}$$

The LCD for 4 and 16 is 16 (16/4 = 4 and 16/16 = 1). The problem can then be written as follows:

$$\frac{13 \times 4}{4 \times 4} + \frac{81 \times 1}{16 \times 1} = \frac{52}{16} + \frac{81}{16}$$

$$= \frac{52 + 81}{16} = \frac{133}{16}$$

Since the solution is an improper fraction, it can be converted into a mixed fraction as follows:

$$= \frac{133}{16} = 8\frac{5}{16}$$

Alternatively, the problem can also be solved by first changing the fractions to contain the same denominators without changing the value of fractions, and then adding them as per the following formula, where A and D are whole numbers:

$$A\frac{B}{C} + D\frac{E}{C} = A + D\frac{B + E}{C}$$

In the above problem, the denominator of each fraction can be changed to 16, and the problem can be written as follows:

$$= 3\frac{1 \times 4}{4 \times 4} + 5\frac{1 \times 1}{16 \times 1} = 3\frac{4}{16} + 5\frac{1}{16}$$

$$= (3+5)\frac{(4+1)}{16} = 8\frac{5}{16}$$

Example 2: Find the sum of:

$$1\frac{1}{2} + 1\frac{3}{4} + \frac{2}{5}$$

The first fraction:

$$1\frac{1}{2} = \frac{(2 \times 1) + 1}{2} = \frac{2+1}{2} = \frac{3}{2}$$

The second fraction:

$$1\frac{3}{4} = \frac{(4 \times 1) + 3}{4} = \frac{4+3}{4} = \frac{7}{4}$$

The third fraction:

$$\frac{2}{5}$$

The LCD for 2, 4, and 5 is 20 (20/2 = 10, 20/4 = 5, and 20/5 = 4). Using this LCD, the problem can be written as follows:

$$= \frac{3 \times 10}{2 \times 10} + \frac{7 \times 5}{4 \times 5} + \frac{2 \times 4}{5 \times 4}$$

$$= \frac{30}{20} + \frac{35}{20} + \frac{8}{20}$$

$$= \frac{30 + 35 + 8}{20} = \frac{73}{20} = 3\frac{13}{20}$$

Alternatively, it can also be solved as follows:

$$=1\frac{1\times 10}{2\times 10}+1\frac{3\times 5}{4\times 5}+\frac{2\times 4}{5\times 4}=1\frac{10}{20}+1\frac{15}{20}+\frac{8}{20}$$

$$=2\frac{10+15+8}{20}=2\frac{33}{20}=2\frac{20+13}{20}=2+\frac{20}{20}+\frac{13}{20}$$

$$=2+1+\frac{13}{20}=3\frac{13}{20}$$

Subtraction of Fractions

To subtract fractions, the following steps may be used:

1. Find a least common denominator (LCD) or the smallest number that is divided by all the denominators evenly.
2. Change each fraction so that it has that denominator but retains its original value.
3. Subtract the numerators.
4. Reduce the resulting fraction to its lowest terms.

Note: The steps for both addition and subtraction of fractions are exactly the same, except in step 3 where the numerators are subtracted instead of added. The general formula for subtraction can be expressed as follows:

$$\boxed{\frac{A}{B}-\frac{C}{B}=\frac{A-C}{B}}$$

Example 1: Find the difference of: $\frac{4}{7}-\frac{3}{7}=\frac{4-3}{7}=\frac{1}{7}$

Complex, multiple subtractions can be performed according to the following expression:

$$\boxed{\frac{A}{B}-\frac{C}{B}-\frac{D}{B}=\frac{A}{B}-\left[\frac{C+D}{B}\right]=\frac{A-(C+D)}{B}}$$

$$\frac{9}{10}-\frac{3}{10}-\frac{1}{10}=\frac{9}{10}-\left[\frac{3+1}{10}\right]$$

$$\frac{9-(3+1)}{10}=\frac{9-4}{10}=\frac{5}{10}=\frac{1}{2}$$

Example 2: Find the difference of: $2\frac{1}{4}-\frac{4}{5}$

The first fraction is a mixed fraction, which should be converted into improper fraction as follows:

$$= 2\frac{1}{4} = \frac{(4 \times 2) + 1}{4} = \frac{9}{4}$$

The subtraction then can be performed as follows:

$$= \frac{9}{4} - \frac{4}{5} = \frac{9 \times 5}{4 \times 5} - \frac{4 \times 4}{5 \times 4}$$

$$= \frac{45}{20} - \frac{16}{20} = \frac{45 - 16}{20} = \frac{29}{20}$$

This improper fraction can then be converted back into a mixed fraction as follows:

$$29/20 = 1\frac{9}{20}$$

Example 3: Find the difference of: $\frac{23}{25} - \frac{1}{5} - \frac{1}{4}$

The LCD for 25, 5, and 4 is 100 (100/25 = 4, 100/5 = 20, and 100/4 = 25), and using this LCD, the problem can be written as:

$$= \frac{23 \times 4}{4 \times 25} - \frac{1 \times 20}{5 \times 20} - \frac{1 \times 25}{4 \times 25}$$

$$= \frac{92}{100} - \left[\frac{20 + 25}{100}\right]$$

$$= \frac{92}{100} - \frac{45}{100}$$

$$= \frac{92 - 45}{100} = \frac{47}{100}$$

The result is a proper fraction and cannot be further reduced.

Multiplication of Fractions

To multiply fractions, the following steps can be used:

1. Multiply the two numerators and the two denominators.

   Example:

$$\frac{3}{4} \times \frac{5}{8} = \frac{3 \times 5}{4 \times 8} = \frac{15}{24}$$

2. Reduce the answer, when possible, to lowest terms by dividing both numerator and denominator with the least common factor (LCF).

$$\text{e.g.,} \frac{15}{24} = \frac{[15/3]}{[24/3]} = \frac{5}{8}$$

3. When possible, divide the numerator of any of the fractions and the denominator of any of the fractions by the same number. Then multiply the numerators and denominators. In such cases no further reduction can be made, since the fraction is already in its lowest terms.

Example: Solve $\frac{3}{9} \times \frac{4}{12}$

First, simplification of the fractions:

First fraction: $\frac{3/3}{9/3} = \frac{1}{3}$

Second fraction: $\frac{4/4}{12/4} = \frac{1}{4}$

Multiply the products of each of the simplified terms.

$$\frac{1}{3} \times \frac{1}{4} = \frac{1 \times 1}{3 \times 4} = \frac{1}{12}$$

4. To multiply a fraction with a whole number, assume the denominator of the whole number to be 1. Then multiply the numerator and denominator in the same way as explained above in step 1.
For example, 5 can be expressed as 5/1.

Example: Find the product of: $30 \times 6\frac{2}{5}$

$$\frac{30}{1} \times \frac{(5 \times 6) + 2}{5} = \frac{30 \times 32}{5}$$

$$= \frac{960}{5} = \frac{960/5}{5/5} = 192$$

5. When there are mixed numbers, use the following steps to solve the problem.
   Change each number to an improper fraction.
   Simplify when possible.
   Multiply the numerators and then the denominators.
   Express the answer in the lowest possible terms.

Example: Find the product of: $4\frac{2}{5} \times \frac{10}{11}$

First, convert the mixed number into an improper fraction:

$$4\frac{2}{5} = \frac{(4 \times 5) + 2}{5} = \frac{20 + 2}{5} = \frac{22}{5}$$

Multiply the fractions:

$$\frac{22}{5} \times \frac{10}{11} = \frac{220}{55}$$

Simplify the product by dividing both numerator and denominator with 55 as follows:

$$\frac{220}{55} = \frac{\left[{}^{220}\!/_{55}\right]}{\left[{}^{55}\!/_{55}\right]} = \frac{4}{1} = 4$$

Remember the following:

1. $\boxed{\frac{0}{A} = 0}$
2. $\boxed{\frac{A}{0} = \infty}$
3. $\boxed{A \times \frac{B}{C} = \frac{A}{1} \times \frac{B}{C} = \frac{A \times B}{C}}$
4. $\boxed{1 \times \frac{A}{B} = \frac{A}{B}}$
5. $\boxed{\frac{A}{B} = \frac{A \times C}{B \times C}}$

Example 1: Solve $\frac{1}{5} \times \frac{2}{3}$

$$\frac{1}{5} \times \frac{2}{3} = \frac{2}{15}$$

Example 2: Solve $\frac{3}{12} \times \frac{4}{4}$

$$\frac{3/3}{12/3} \times \frac{4}{4} = \frac{1}{4} \times \frac{4}{4} = \frac{4}{16}$$

$$= \frac{4/4}{16/4} = \frac{1}{4}$$

Example 3: $5\frac{2}{3} \times \frac{1}{4}$

First, convert the mixed number into an improper fraction:

$$5\frac{2}{3} = \frac{(5 \times 3) + 2}{3} = \frac{15 + 2}{3} = \frac{17}{3}$$

Multiply the fractions:

$$\frac{17}{3} \times \frac{1}{4} = \frac{17}{12}$$

17/12 can be further reduced to a mixed fraction as $1\frac{5}{12}$

Division of Fractions

Division of any number by a fraction is similar to multiplying fractions, except for one additional step.

1. Multiply the number by the reciprocal of the fraction.
2. Simplify the resulting fraction if possible.
3. Multiply the result with the divisor. This value should be equal to the original dividend.

Note. Only non-zero fractions can be divided. In the division of fractions, the following terms should be recognized:

$$\boxed{\frac{A}{B} = C = \frac{Dividend}{Divisor} = Quotient}$$

Dividend (A) = The number to be divided.
Divisor (B) = The number by which the dividend is divided.
Quotient (C) = The number obtained by dividing the dividend with the devisor.
Dividend ÷ divisor = quotient; this expression may be read as "dividend is divided by divisor to obtain the quotient."

Note the following:

$$\boxed{\frac{A}{B} \div \frac{C}{D} = \frac{A}{B} \times \frac{D}{C}}$$

Whole numbers are assumed to have a denominator of 1.

When there is a mixed number in the problem, first change it to an improper function, invert the divisor, and then multiply.

Example 1: Find the quotient of: $\frac{1}{2} \div \frac{1}{4}$

$$\frac{1}{2} \times \frac{4}{1} = \frac{(1 \times 4)}{(2 \times 1)} = \frac{4}{2} = 2$$

Example 2: Find the quotient of: $\frac{6}{8} \div \frac{9}{14}$

$$= \frac{6}{8} \times \frac{14}{9} = \frac{(6 \times 14)}{(8 \times 9)}$$

$$= \frac{84}{72} \text{ or}$$

$$= \frac{7}{6} = 1\frac{1}{6}, \text{ answer}$$

Example 3: Find the quotient of: $8 \div 5\frac{1}{2}$

$$= 8 \div 5\frac{1}{2} = 8 \div \frac{(2 \times 5) + 1}{2}$$

$$= \frac{8}{1} \div \frac{11}{2}$$

$$= \frac{8}{1} \times \frac{2}{11}$$

$$= \frac{8 \times 2}{1 \times 11} = \frac{16}{11} = 1\frac{5}{11}, \text{ answer}$$

Example 4: Find the quotient of: $15\frac{1}{2} \div 5\frac{3}{4}$

$$= 15\frac{1}{2} \div 5\frac{3}{4} = \frac{31}{2} \div \frac{23}{4} = \frac{31}{\cancel{2}_1} \times \frac{4^2}{23} = \frac{31 \times 2}{1 \times 23}$$

$$= \frac{62}{23} = \frac{62/_{23}}{23/_{23}} = 2\frac{16}{23}, \textit{ answer}$$

DECIMALS

Decimals are another means of expressing a fractional amount. A decimal is a fraction whose denominator is 10 or a multiple of 10.

Examples:

0.7 = 7/10
0.06 = 6/100
0.008 = 8/1000

A *decimal mixed number* is a whole number and a decimal fraction.

Example:

4.3 = 4(3/10)

Each position to the left of the decimal is ten times the previous place, and each position to the right is one-tenth the previous place. The position to the left or right of the decimal point is referred to as place value, which determines the size of the denominator. Figure 2.1 indicates the place value of the numerals to the left and right of the decimal point.

Adding zeros to a decimal that do not change the place value of the numerals does not affect the value of the number. However, adding or subtracting zeros between the decimal point and the numeral does change the value of the number.

Example:

0.2, 0.20, or 0.200; all these represent two-tenths
But, 0.2 = two-tenths
0.02 = two-hundredths
0.002 = two-thousandths

Addition and Subtraction

In order to add or subtract decimals, all the numbers are lined up so that all numbers with the same place value are in the same column. Then perform addition or subtraction.

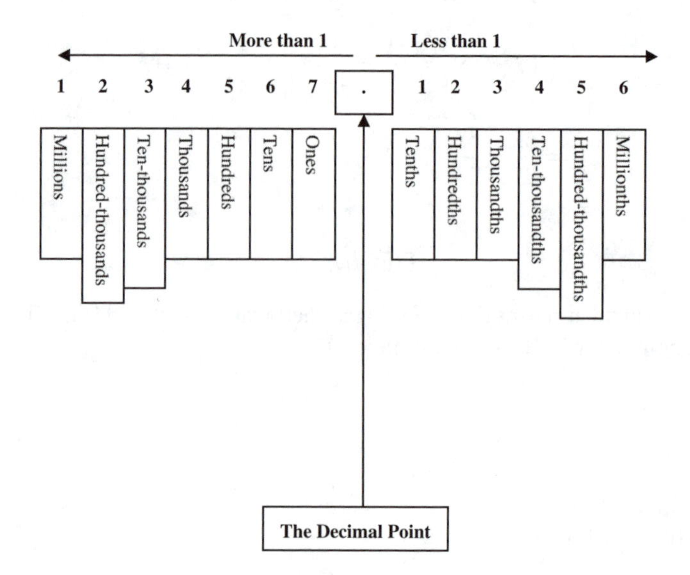

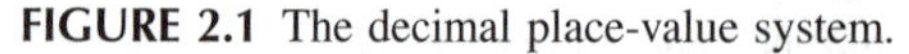

FIGURE 2.1 The decimal place-value system.

Examples:

Addition:

$$\begin{array}{r} 16.24 \\ 8.12 \\ \underline{+12.62} \\ 36.98 \end{array}$$

Subtraction:

$$\begin{array}{r} 43.78 \\ \underline{-8.43} \\ 35.35 \end{array}$$

Multiplication

To multiply decimals, multiply the numerals as usual and move the decimal point in the answer to the left by as many places as there are in the sum of the decimal places in the two numbers being multiplied.

Example:

8.23×6.76 (sum of the decimal places in the two numbers is 4)

$823 \times 676 = 556348$

55.6348

Division

To divide decimals, the following steps may be used:

1. Change the divisor to a whole number by moving the decimal point to the right.
2. Move the decimal point in the dividend to the right by the same number of places.
3. Divide.
4. Place the decimal point in the quotient above the decimal in the dividend.

Example:

Divide 26 by 2.006
Change the divisor and dividend to whole numbers by moving the decimal point to the right:

Dividend = 26000
Divisor = 2006

Divide.

```
        12.961
        ————
2006.  26000.000
       2006
        ——
        5940
        4012
        ——
        1928 0
        1805 4
        ——
         122 60
         120 36
          ——
          2 240
          2 006
          ——
           234
```

PRACTICE PROBLEMS

Solve the following problems:

1. $2\frac{1}{4}+3\frac{1}{2}$
2. $\frac{1}{6}+\frac{1}{3}+\frac{1}{2}$
3. $\frac{1}{8}+\frac{1}{3}$
4. $7\frac{1}{6}+\frac{5}{6}$
5. $6+3\frac{4}{5}$
6. $12\frac{7}{8}+13$
7. $5\frac{12}{15}+3\frac{1}{5}+6\frac{1}{3}$
8. $8\frac{1}{2}+15\frac{1}{2}$
9. $5\frac{1}{2}+3\frac{1}{4}+2\frac{1}{8}$
10. $8\frac{1}{3}+\frac{7}{9}+11\frac{5}{6}$
11. $\frac{3}{4}-\frac{1}{2}$
12. $\frac{8}{9}-\frac{7}{11}$
13. $3\frac{1}{8}-1\frac{1}{4}$
14. $\frac{25}{3}+3\frac{1}{2}$
15. $9\frac{1}{7}-\frac{23}{5}$
16. $8-7\frac{1}{2}$
17. $19\frac{1}{5}-\frac{3}{4}-2\frac{2}{5}$
18. $20\frac{1}{2}-7\frac{1}{3}-11\frac{7}{11}$
19. $22-11\frac{1}{3}-2\frac{1}{2}$
20. $56-24\frac{1}{5}$
21. $\frac{1}{2}\times\frac{1}{4}$
22. $\frac{3}{9}\times\frac{2}{5}$
23. $\frac{4}{7}\times\frac{2}{3}\times\frac{3}{4}$
24. $3\frac{1}{2}\times4\frac{1}{3}\times2$
25. $\frac{3}{4}\times\frac{2}{3}$
26. $\frac{5}{8}\times\frac{4}{10}$
27. $14\frac{1}{9}\times2\frac{1}{4}$
28. $3\frac{1}{9}\times8\frac{1}{10}\times\frac{20}{7}$
29. $\frac{16}{9}\times\frac{36}{64}$
30. $1\frac{2}{3}\times2\frac{1}{2}\times\frac{6}{15}\times5$
31. $3\div\frac{1}{4}$
32. $3\div\frac{3}{4}$
33. $\frac{1}{3}\div\frac{3}{4}$
34. $\frac{5}{7}\div\frac{10}{15}$
35. $8\div\frac{1}{16}$
36. $\frac{16}{25}\div16$

37. $7 \div \frac{1}{7}$

38. $30\frac{1}{2} \div 610$

39. $150 \div 1\frac{1}{2}$

40. $820 \div 2\frac{1}{2}$

41. $\frac{3}{10} + \frac{2}{5} + \frac{6}{15}$

42. $1\frac{1}{3} + 6\frac{1}{5} + \frac{4}{5}$

43. $22\frac{1}{8} + 41\frac{1}{5} + 36\frac{9}{20}$

44. $3\frac{1}{2} + 8\frac{1}{2} + 9\frac{1}{4} + 12\frac{1}{6} + 7$

45. $8\frac{3}{4} - \frac{17}{24}$

46. $12\frac{1}{7} - 2\frac{1}{3}$

47. $0 \times 22\frac{1}{2}$

48. $2\frac{1}{2} \times 2\frac{1}{2} \times 2\frac{1}{2} \times 2\frac{1}{2}$

49. $16 \div 1\frac{1}{2}$

50. $3\frac{1}{3} \div 3\frac{1}{3}$

51. What is the total weight of 25 capsules when each capsule weighs $\frac{4}{5}$ grain?
52. A bottle contains 60 mL of syrup. If one dose is $\frac{3}{4}$ mL, how many doses can this bottle provide?
53. How many $\frac{1}{2}$-grain capsules can be prepared from 25 grains of a powder medication?
54. If each dose is 2.5 mL, how many doses are contained in 50 mL?
55. If each capsule weighs $\frac{4}{5}$ grain, a third of which ($\frac{1}{3}$) is the capsule shell weight, what will be the total weight of powder in 25 capsules?
56. Simplify the following fractions:
    a. 12/24
    b. 6/9
    c. 18/10
    d. 10/9
57. Convert the following mixed numbers to their corresponding improper fractions:
    a. $2\frac{3}{4}$
    b. $1\frac{1}{2}$
    c. $11\frac{7}{10}$
    d. $9\frac{1}{10}$
58. A pharmacist mixed 1 g of ingredient A, $\frac{1}{2}$ g of ingredient B, and $1\frac{4}{5}$ g of ingredient C. What is the total weight of this mixture?
59. If each tablet weighs $\frac{3}{4}$ g, what will be the total weight of 24 tablets?
60. A container with some pills weighs 34 grams. If 80 pills, weighing $\frac{1}{4}$ g each are removed from it, what will be the final weight of the container with the remaining pills?
61. A pharmacist mixed $1\frac{1}{4}$ g of ingredient A, $\frac{2}{3}$ g of ingredient B and $\frac{1}{12}$ g of ingredient C. If he weighs out $1\frac{1}{2}$ g of the mixture, how much of the mixture will be left?

62. A bottle contains 30 mL of syrup. If one dose is ½ mL, how many doses can this bottle provide?
63. In a mixture, ½ portion is ingredient A, ⅓ portion is ingredient B, 1⁄12 portion is ingredient C and the rest is ingredient D, what will be the amount of ingredient D if the total weight of the mixture is 2400 mg?
64. A medication order calls for 20 tablets, each containing ¾ grain of a certain medication. If 10 grains of this medication is available, how much extra medication is needed to fill this prescription?
65. How many capsules containing ½ grain of medication can be prepared from 35½ grains of this medication powder?
66. If a patient is required to take ½ teaspoonful of a syrup 4 times a day, and if he has to continue the prescription for 4 weeks, how many bottles of syrup does he need to purchase if each bottle contains 30 teaspoonfuls of syrup?
67. A pharmacy technician accidentally dropped half the medication from a bottle that contained 20 teaspoonfuls of a pediatric cough syrup. How many ½-teaspoonful doses are still left in the bottle?
68. What will be the total amount of medication in grains if 45 capsules, each containing ⅗ grain, are dispensed?
69. How many ⅔ g tablets can be prepared from a stock of 66 g?
70. If each capsule containing certain powder medication weighs ⅗ grain, of which ⅓ portion is the capsule shell, what will be the total weight of powder in 25 capsules?
71. When 11⅓ g of powder A, 25 g of powder B, 2 1⁄15 g of powder C, and 3⅖ g of powder D are mixed together, what will be the total weight of the mixture?
72. How many doses are contained in 55 mL, if each dose is 5 mL?
73. If a soft gelatin capsule contains 4¼ mL of cod liver oil, what will be the total dose if 20 such capsules are taken?
74. If 12 doses of 1½ mL are taken from a bottle that contains 40 mL, what will be the remaining quantity?
75. If there is only a 6 3⁄2 mL measuring cylinder available to fill a 105-mL bottle, how many times will it be used to measure the desired amount of liquid?
76. What is the total volume of daily dose if the prescription says 2½ mL of syrup A, 4 times per day?
77. A prescription calls for 1½ milliliters, 3 times a day for 2 weeks. How many such prescriptions can be filled from a stock of 2.52 liters?
78. What will be the total weight when 25¾ g of ingredient A is mixed with 2¼ g of ingredient B?
79. If a multivitamin-syrup contains ½ mg of riboflavin, ¾ mg of niacin, ⅗ mg of pyridoxine and ⅙ mg ascorbic acid, what is the total amount of vitamin in this preparation?
80. If a 6-mL soft gelatin capsule contains 2¾ mL of vitamin A and the remaining volume is vitamin D, what will be the total volume of vitamin D in 20 capsules?

ANSWERS

1. $5\frac{3}{4}$
2. 1
3. $\frac{11}{24}$
4. 8
5. $9\frac{4}{5}$
6. $25\frac{7}{8}$
7. $15\frac{1}{3}$
8. 24
9. $10\frac{7}{8}$
10. $20\frac{17}{18}$
11. $\frac{1}{4}$
12. $\frac{25}{99}$
13. $1\frac{7}{8}$
14. $11\frac{5}{6}$
15. $4\frac{19}{35}$
16. $\frac{1}{2}$
17. $16\frac{1}{20}$
18. $1\frac{35}{66}$
19. $8\frac{1}{6}$
20. $31\frac{4}{5}$
21. $\frac{1}{8}$
22. $\frac{2}{15}$
23. $\frac{2}{7}$
24. $30\frac{1}{3}$
25. $\frac{1}{2}$
26. $\frac{1}{4}$
27. $31\frac{3}{4}$
28. 72
29. 1
30. $8\frac{1}{3}$
31. 12
32. 4
33. $\frac{4}{9}$
34. $1\frac{1}{14}$
35. 128
36. $\frac{1}{25}$
37. 49
38. $\frac{1}{20}$
39. 100
40. 328
41. $1\frac{1}{10}$
42. $8\frac{1}{3}$
43. $99\frac{31}{40}$
44. $40\frac{5}{12}$
45. $8\frac{1}{24}$
46. $9\frac{17}{21}$
47. 0
48. $39\frac{1}{16}$
49. $10\frac{2}{3}$
50. 1
51. 20 gr
52. 80
53. 50
54. 20
55. 13.33 gr
56. a. 1/2
    b. 2/3
    c. $1\frac{4}{5}$
    d. $1\frac{1}{9}$
57. a. 11/4
    b. 3/2
    c. 111/10
    d. 91/10
58. $3\frac{3}{10}$ g
59. 18 g
60. 14 g
61. $\frac{1}{2}$ g
62. 60
63. 200 mg
64. 5 gr
65. 71
66. 2
67. 20
68. 27 gr
69. 99
70. 10 gr
71. $41\frac{4}{5}$ g

72. 11
73. 85 mL
74. 22 mL
75. 14
76. 10 mL
77. 40
78. 28 g
79. $2\frac{1}{60}$ mg
80. 65 mL

3 Using Ratios, Proportions, and Percentages in Dosage Calculations

Calculations involving ratios, proportions, and percentages are very important in the dispensing and compounding of medications. Following is a discussion on these topics, followed by a variety of practice problems highlighting some of the important applications of ratios, proportions, and percentage calculations.

RATIOS

A ratio is a comparison of two numbers or like quantities. A colon (:) generally separates the two numbers in a ratio. For example, the ratio of 8 and 12 can be written as 8:12 or as a fraction 8/12, and it can be expressed as *eight to twelve*. A ratio, therefore, is the relation in degree or number between two similar things. The relation between two quantities can also be expressed as a quotient, where one quantity is divided by the other. For example, the ratio of 9 to 5 can be written as 9/5. A ratio can also be expressed as a percentage or a decimal.

Definitions at a Glance

Quotient A quotient is the number obtained by dividing one quantity by another. For example, $30 \div 3 = 10$; the answer 10 is the quotient.

Fraction A fraction is an expression that indicates the quotient of two quantities, such as 1/3. Other ways of expressing this fraction include 1:3 or 1 is to 3.

Decimal A decimal is another way of expressing a fractional amount and has a denominator of 10 or 10^x ($x \geq 1$). For example, 0.15 = 15/100 = 15:100 or 15 is to 100.

A ratio can therefore be used to compare two different things. For example, someone can look at a group of people, measure their heights, and refer to the "ratio of men to women" in that group. Suppose there are forty-five people, twenty of whom are men. Then the ratio of men to women in this group is 20 to 25.

PROPORTIONS

Two equal fractions can be written as proportion. A proportion is an equation with a ratio on each side. It is a statement that two ratios are equal. An example of a proportion is 3/4 = 6/8. Other forms to express proportions are as follows:

a:b::c:d

a:b = c:d

a/b = c/d

When one of the four numbers in a proportion is unknown, cross products may be used to find the unknown number. This is called solving the proportion. A proportion, when written as 1/2 = 5/10, can be read as "one is to two as five is to ten," and 8/16 = 22/44 may be read as "8 is to 16 as 22 is to 44."

Multiplying or dividing each term by the same number (except zero) will not change the value of the ratio. For example, the ratio of 30:6 (or 30/6) has a value of 5. If both terms are multiplied by 3, the ratio becomes 90:18 (or 90/18) and still has the same value of 5. Similarly, if both terms are divided by 3 or 6, the resulting ratios 10:2 and 5:1 still have the same value of 5.

Ratios having the same values are equivalent. Cross products of two equivalent ratios are equal, i.e., the product of the numerator of first fraction and the denominator of the second fraction always equals the product of the denominator of the first fraction and the numerator of the second fraction. For example, ratios 3:4 and 6:8 are equal, because their cross products ($3 \times 8 = 4 \times 6$) are equal.

Note: If the two ratios are equal, their reciprocals will also be equal.

If $\frac{a}{b} = \frac{c}{d}$

then, $\frac{b}{a} = \frac{d}{c}$

other forms of expression:

$$a = \frac{b \times c}{d}$$

or:

$$b = \frac{a \times d}{c}$$

For example, 3/4 = 6/8 (a/b = c/d).

$$\frac{4}{3} = 1\frac{1}{3} = \frac{8}{6} = 1\frac{2}{6}$$

When solving for a or b, we can write them as follows:

$$a = \frac{b \times c}{d} \text{ or } 3 = \frac{4 \times 6}{8} = \frac{24}{8}$$

$$b = \frac{a \times d}{c} \quad or \quad 4 = \frac{3 \times 8}{6} = \frac{24}{6}$$

Find the products of the following and express the results as ratios in different ways:

Example 1: $4 \div 8$

$$\frac{4}{1} \div \frac{8}{1} = \frac{4}{1} \times \frac{1}{8} = \frac{4}{8} = \frac{1}{2}$$

As a ratio, the product can be expressed as:

Fraction: $\frac{1}{2}$

Percentage: $\frac{1}{2} \times 100 = 50\%$

Decimal: $\frac{1}{2} \times \frac{5}{5} = \frac{5}{10} = 0.5$

Note: To write the product as decimal, we shall multiply or divide both the numerator and denominator by a number (whole number, mixed number or fraction) that turn the denominator into 10. In Example 1, both numerator and denominator are multiplied with 5.

Example 2: $3\frac{1}{3} \div 5$

$$\frac{(3 \times 3) + 1}{3} \div \frac{5}{1} = \frac{10}{3} \times \frac{1}{5} = \frac{10}{15} = \frac{2}{3}$$

As a ratio, the product can be expressed as:

Fraction: $\frac{2}{3}$

Percentage: $\frac{2}{3} \times 100 = 66.66\%$

Decimal: $\frac{2}{3} \times \frac{3.33}{3.33} = \frac{6.66}{10} = 0.666$

Example 3: $2\frac{1}{7} \div 15$

$$\frac{(7 \times 2) + 1}{7} \div \frac{15}{1} = \frac{15}{7} \times \frac{1}{15} = \frac{15 \times 1}{7 \times 15} = \frac{1}{7}$$

As a ratio, the product can be expressed as:

Fraction: $\frac{1}{7}$

Percentage: $\frac{1}{7} \times 100 = 14.29\%$

Decimal: $\frac{1}{7} \times \frac{1.43}{1.43} = \frac{1.43}{10} = 0.143$

Example 4: $10\frac{1}{4} \div 5\frac{1}{2}$

$$\frac{(4 \times 10) + 1}{4} \div \frac{(2 \times 5) + 1}{2} = \frac{41}{4^2} \times \frac{\cancel{2}^1}{11} = \frac{41}{22} = 1\frac{19}{22}$$

As a ratio, the product can be expressed as:

Fraction: $\frac{41}{22}$

Percentage: $\frac{41}{22} \times 100 = 186.36\%$

Decimal: $\frac{41 \div 2.2}{22 \div 2.2} = \frac{18.63}{10} = 1.863$

Example 5: Find the missing number in the proportion: $\frac{2}{3} = \frac{x}{12}$

$$3x = 2 \times 12$$

$$x = \frac{2 \times \cancel{12}^4}{3^1} = \frac{8}{1} = 8$$

$$\therefore \frac{2}{3} = \frac{8}{12}$$

Example 6: Find the missing denominator in the proportion: $\frac{2}{3} = \frac{12}{x}$

$$2x = 3 \times 12$$

$$x = \frac{3 \times \cancel{12}^6}{\cancel{2}^1} = \frac{18}{1} = 18$$

$$\therefore \frac{2}{3} = \frac{12}{18}$$

Proportions are routinely used in dosage calculations. For example, to find out how many milligrams of the drug acetaminophen is present in 5 milliliters (mL) when there are 50 mg of acetaminophen in each mL, a proportion can be set as:

$$\therefore \frac{1(mL)}{5(mL)} = \frac{15(mg)}{x(mg)}$$

$$x = \frac{5 \times 15}{1} = 75\ mg$$

Example 7: What is the percentage strength (w/v) of sodium chloride solution, if 600 mL contain 150 g?

$$\therefore \frac{150(g)}{x(g)} = \frac{600(mL)}{100(mL)}$$

$$x = \frac{150 \times 100}{600} = \frac{150}{6} = 25$$

25 g in 100 mL is 25%

Example 8: What is the percentage strength (w/v) of a urea solution, if 90 mL contain 18 g?

Note. 90 mL of water weigh 90 g.

$$\therefore \frac{90(g)}{18(g)} = \frac{100(\%)}{x(\%)}$$

$$x = \frac{100 \times \not{18}^{1}}{\not{90}^{5}} = \frac{100}{5} = 20\%$$

Example 9: How many milliliters of a 7% atropine sulfate solution in water can be prepared from 28 g of atropine sulfate?

$$\therefore \frac{7(g)}{100(mL)} = \frac{28(g)}{x(mL)}$$

$$x = \frac{100 \times \not{28}^{4}}{\not{7}^{1}} = \frac{400}{1} = 400\ mL$$

Example 10: How many grams of iodine should be used in preparing 50 mL of 2:100 and 5:100 solutions?

Method 1:

Amount of iodine needed to prepare 50 mL of 2:100 solution:

$$2{:}100 = 2\ g\ in\ 100\ mL\ of\ solution$$

$$\frac{100(mL)}{50(mL)} = \frac{2(g)}{x(g)}$$

$$x = \frac{50 \times 2}{100} = 1.0\ g$$

Amount of iodine needed for 50 mL of 5:100 solution:

$$5{:}100 = 5\ g\ in\ 100\ mL\ of\ solution$$

$$\frac{100(mL)}{50(mL)} = \frac{5(g)}{x(g)}$$

$$x = \frac{50 \times 5}{100} = 2.5\ g$$

Method 2:

Amount of iodine needed for 50 mL of 2:100 solution:

$$\because 2{:}100 = 2\%$$

$$\therefore 50\ g \times \frac{2}{100} = 1\ g$$

Amount of iodine needed for 50 mL of 5:100 solution:

$$\because 5{:}100 = 5\%$$

$$\therefore 50\ g \times \frac{5}{100} = 2.5\ g$$

Use of proportions is very common in dosage calculations, especially in finding out the drug concentration per teaspoonful or in the preparation of bulk or stock solutions of certain medications. In a given proportion, when any three terms are known, the missing term can be determined. Thus, for example, if a/b = c/d, then a = bc/d, or any other term can be calculated from the other three known terms (see page 28).

For example, to find out how many milligrams of the drug Demerol is present in 5 mL when there are 15 mg of Demerol in 1 mL, a proportion can be set as:

drug:volume = drug:volume

15 mg:1 mL = X mg:5 mL

X = 15 × 5 = 75 mg

Example 11: If 4 g of sucrose are dissolved in enough water to make 250 mL, what is the concentration in terms of % w/v of the solution?

By the method of proportion:

$$4 \text{ g} \div 250 \text{ mL} = \text{X g} \div 100 \text{ mL}$$

Solving for X, we get:

$$\text{X} = (100 \times 4) \div 250 = 1.6 \text{ g}$$

1.6 g in 100 mL is 1.6% w/v, answer

Example 12: An injection contains 40 mg pentobarbital sodium in each mL of solution. What is the concentration in terms of % w/v of this solution?

By the method of proportion:

$$40 \text{ mg} \div 1 \text{ mL} = \text{X mg} \div 100 \text{ mL}$$

Solving for X, we get:

$$\text{X} = (100 \times 40) = 4000 \text{ mg or } 4 \text{ g}$$

4 g in 100 mL is 4% w/v, answer

Example 13: How many grams of zinc chloride should be used in preparing 5 liters of the mouthwash containing 1/10% w/v of zinc chloride?

$$1/10\% = 0.1\% = 0.1 \text{ g in } 100 \text{ mL}$$

By the method of proportion:

$$0.1 \text{ g} \div 100 \text{ mL} = \text{X g} \div 5000 \text{ mL}$$

$$\text{X} = (0.1 \times 5000)/100$$

$$\text{X} = 5.0 \text{ g, answer}$$

PRACTICE PROBLEMS

Ratios and Proportions

Solve the following problems and express the results in terms of ratios as fractions, decimals, and percentages:

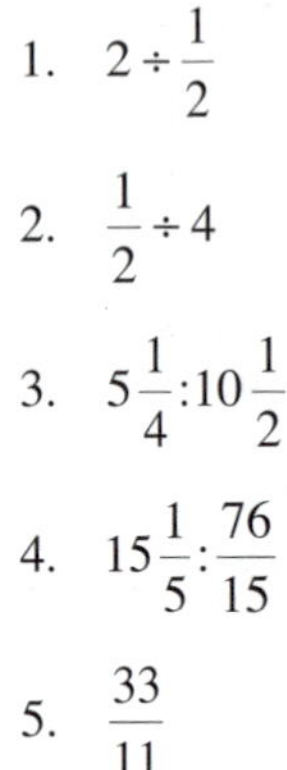

1. $2 \div \frac{1}{2}$
2. $\frac{1}{2} \div 4$
3. $5\frac{1}{4}:10\frac{1}{2}$
4. $15\frac{1}{5}:\frac{76}{15}$
5. $\frac{33}{11}$
6. $3\frac{5}{9} \div 7\frac{1}{5}$
7. How many grams of potassium permanganate should be used in preparing 300 mL of a $\frac{1}{2}$:1250 solution?
8. How many milligrams of iodine should be used to prepare 50 mL of 2:100 iodine solution, and if potassium iodide should be added in a ratio of 2:1 to get a soluble form of iodine, how many milligrams of potassium iodide are needed to prepare such prescription?
9. How many grams of sodium chloride should be used in preparing of 500 mL of a 1:25 solution?
10. A nurse was instructed to give a dehydrated patient 500 mL of 25% dextrose and 1000 mL of 0.9% saline as intravenous infusion. What is the ratio between volumes of dextrose to saline ordered for this patient?
11. If the dose of a drug, misoprostol, is 100 micrograms, how many doses are contained in 0.5 grams?
12. If a tablet containing 10 milligrams torsemide is to be taken twice a day, how many grams of torsemide will a patient consume in 2 months?
13. If a cough syrup contains 150 mg of codeine in 200 milliliters, how many milligrams of codeine are contained in 30 milliliters?
14. If a cough syrup contains 120 milligrams of codeine in 250 mL, how many milligrams of codeine are contained in 15 milliliters?
15. If a dose of an experimental drug for a patient weighing 132 lbs is ⅓ mg/kg of body weight, taken 3 times a day for 10 days, how many 20-mg tablets of this product should be dispensed?
16. If a patient has been instructed to take 5 milliliters of sulfamethoxazole oral suspension containing 100 mg/mL every 8 hours, how many days will a 5-fluid-ounce (150 milliliters) bottle of the suspension last?
17. A physician prescribed primidone oral suspension for an epileptic patient to be taken in doses of 10 milliliters 4 times a day for 15 days. If the concentration of this suspension is 50 mg/mL, how many milligrams of the drug will the patient receive in 15 days?

18. Griseofulvin oral suspension contains 125 mg/5 mL. How many grams of this drug are contained in 2.5 liters?
19. Simethicone oral suspension contains 40 mg/0.6 milliliters. How many grams of this drug are contained in 0.15 liters?
20. A physician prescribed gentamycin antibiotic for a patient to be administered on the basis of the body weight. If the prescription reads "2 mg/kg, once a day, 10 days," and if the patient weights 140.8 lbs, what will be the total amount (in mg) of gentamycin this patient receives?
21. Hibiclens skin cleanser solution contains 4 g of chlorhexidine gluconate in 100 mL. If 0.25 mL of this product is used 4 times a day, how many milligrams of chlorhexidine gluconate are represented in volume of this solution used per day?
22. How many milliliters of an injection containing 20 mg of gentamycin in every 2 milliliters should be used in filling a medication order for 5 mg of gentamycin to be administered intramuscularly?
23. If Pepto-Bismol suspension contains 262 mg of bismuth subsalicylate per 15 mL, how many grams of this drug will be contained in 3 liters of this suspension?
24. The dose of a drug is 120 microgram per kg of bodyweight. How many milligrams should be given to a patient weighing 187 lb?
25. The adult dose of a sedative drug in a solution form is 0.04 mL per kg of body weight, to be administered as a single dose. How many milliliters should be administered to a person weighing 143 lb?
26. If a patient's new prescription shows a 20% increase in total dose of the drug, how many milligrams of the drug should the patient take each day now? Assume that the previous daily dose was 200 mg.
27. How many milligrams of metronidazole are represented in 5 mL of 10% w/v syrup?
28. If you need to prepare 20 500-mg tablets, what fraction of a 1-kg stock would you need to use?
29. If 5 mL of a decongestant syrup contains 5 mg of chlorpheniramine maleate, how many mL of this syrup will contain 100 mg of chlorpheniramine maleate?
30. If 1 g of a finely divided charcoal powder can remove 30 mg of a toxin from the stomach, how much charcoal powder should be used for a patient who swallowed 75 mg of toxin?
31. If a physician prescribes 1.2 g of amoxicillin per day for a patient, how many 400-mg capsules should this patient take daily?
32. A patient was taking 500 mg of certain antibiotic. If the requirement for this antibiotic is increased by 50% for this patient, how many milligrams of this drug should the patient take?
33. If an ophthalmic solution contains 2 mg of pilocarpine in each milliliter of solution, how many milliliters of this solution are needed to deliver 0.1 mg of pilocarpine?
34. If normal saline contains 0.9% w/v of sodium chloride, how many kilograms of sodium chloride are needed to prepare 500 liter of normal saline?

35. If a prescription requires a patient to take 100-mg tablets 3 times a day for 1 week, how many similar prescriptions can be filled from a stock containing 420 tablets?
36. How many milliliters of a 20% w/v solution are required to prepare 2 liters of 0.5% w/v solution?
37. If a retail pharmacy fills 200 prescriptions a day with two pharmacists, how many more pharmacists are required to fill 500 prescriptions per day?
38. How many milliliters of 2% (w/v) solution contain the same amount of drug as in 150 mL of 0.1% solution?
39. How many 5 mg tablets of hyoscine can be prepared from 3 grams of hyoscine?
40. If a pediatric expectorant formulation has strength of 0.1% w/v of drug, how many milligrams are represented in 5 milliliters of this formulation?
41. How many milligrams are represented in 275 milliliters of 0.2% (w/v) syrup?
42. How many liters of 0.15% (w/v) solution can be prepared from 3 g of drug?

PERCENTAGE

The word *percent* means "hundredths of a whole," "by the hundred," or "in a hundred" and is represented by the symbol (%). Therefore, 1% is the same as the fraction 1/100 or the decimal fraction 0.01. The word *percentage* indicates "rate per hundred," and represents "parts per 100 parts." A percentage may also be expressed as a ratio or given as a fraction or decimal fraction. For example, 15% indicates 15 parts of 100 parts and may also be expressed as 15/100 or 0.15. A fraction or ratio with 100 is understood as the denominator; for example, 0.98 equals a percentage of 98 (i.e., 98%).

Example:

$$5\% = \frac{5}{100} = \frac{1}{20}$$

To express a percent as a decimal, note that percent means division by 100; with decimals, division by 100 is accomplished by moving the decimal point two places to the left.

Examples:

$$25\% = \frac{25}{100} = \frac{1}{4} = 0.25$$

$$10\% = \frac{10}{100} = \frac{1}{10} = 0.1$$

Converting a Fraction to a Percent

To convert a fraction to a percent, carry out the steps as in the following example:

Convert $\frac{3}{4}$ to a percent.

Divide the numerator of the fraction by the denominator.

$$3 \div 4 = 0.75$$

Note. If the number is already presented as a decimal, complete the steps as follows: Multiply by 100 (move the decimal point two places to the right). Round the answer to the desired precision if necessary, and place (%) sign next to the numeric value.

$$0.75 \times 100 = 75\%$$

Converting a Percent to a Fraction

To convert a percent to a fraction, carry out the steps as in the example shown below.

Convert 80% to a fraction.

Remove the percent sign to be 80.

Make a fraction with the percent as the numerator and 100 as the denominator as: $\frac{80}{100}$

Reduce the fraction to its lowest possible term, if needed, as: $\frac{80}{100} = \frac{4}{5}$

Converting a Decimal to a Percent

To convert a decimal to a percent, carry out the steps as in the following example:

Convert 0.65 to a percent.

Multiply the decimal by 100, and add a percent sign after the number:

$$0.65 \times 100 = 65\%$$

Converting a Percent to a Decimal

To convert a decimal to a percent, drop the percent sign and then divide the numerator by 100.

Examples:

$$0.15\% = \frac{0.15}{100} = \frac{15}{10000} = 0.0015$$

$$45\% = \frac{45}{100} = 0.45$$

Determining Percentage

How much is X as a percent of Y?

$$\frac{X}{Y} \times 100 = Z\%$$

Example: How much is 68 as a percent of 87?

Divide the first number (portion) by the second number (total) as follows:

$$68 \div 87 = 0.7816$$

Multiply the answer by 100 (Move decimal point two places to the right).

$$0.7816 \times 100 = 78.16$$

Round to the desired precision; 78.16 rounded to the nearest whole number = 78.

$$\therefore 68 = 78\% \text{ of } 87$$

Fractions and Equivalent Decimals

A decimal is a type of fractional number. The decimal 0.5 represents the fraction 5/10. The decimal 0.25 represents the fraction 25/100. Decimal fractions always have a denominator based on a power of 10. We know that 5/10 is equivalent to 1/2 since 1/2 times 5/5 is 5/10. Therefore, the decimal 0.5 is equivalent to 1/2 or 2/4.

Some common Equivalent Decimals and Fractions are shown below:

0.1 and 1/10
0.2 and 1/5
0.25 and ¼
0.50 and ½
0.75 and ¾
1.0 and 1/1 or 2/2 or 1

Converting a Fraction to a Decimal

Divide the numerator of the fraction by the denominator, and round the answer to the desired precision as needed.

Convert 4/9 to a decimal.

$$4 \div 9 = 0.4444$$

PERCENT CONCENTRATION EXPRESSIONS

The concentration of a solution may be expressed in terms of the quantity of solute in a definite volume of solution or as the quantity of solute in a definite weight of solution. The quantity (or amount) is an absolute value (e.g., 10 mL, 5 g, 5 mg, etc.), whereas concentration is the quantity of a substance in relation to a definite volume or weight of other substance (e.g., 2 g/5 g, 4 mL/5 mL, 5 mg/1 mL, etc.).

Percent Weight-in-Volume (% *w/v*)

It is the number of grams of a constituent (solute) in 100 milliliters of liquid preparation (solution).

Percent Weight-in-Weight (Percent by Weight), (% *w/w*)

It is the number of grams of a constituent (solute) in 100 grams of preparation (solution).

Percent Volume-in-Volume (Percent by Volume), (% *v/v*)

It is the number of milliliters of a constituent (solute) in 100 milliliters of preparation (solution).

Milligram Percent, (*mg*%)

It is the number of milligrams of a constituent (solute) in 100 milliliters of preparation (solution).

Example 1: How many grams of dextrose should be used to prepare 500 mL of 5% solution?

$$\frac{5(g)}{100(ml)} = \frac{x(g)}{500(ml)}$$

$$x = \frac{5 \times 500}{100} = 25\,g\ dextrose$$

Example 2: How many grams of sodium chloride should be used to prepare a liter of 0.9% solution?

$$\frac{0.9(g)}{100(ml)} = \frac{x(g)}{1000(ml)}$$

$$x = \frac{0.9 \times 1000}{100} = \frac{900}{100}$$

$$= 9.0\,g\ sodium\ chloride$$

Example 3. How many milligrams of gentian violet should be used in preparing: (a) 500 mL 0.001% and (b) 500 mL of 0.003% solution?

$$0.001\% = \frac{1}{100 \times 1000} = \frac{1}{100,000}$$

$$0.003\% = \frac{3}{100 \times 1000} = \frac{3}{100,000}$$

$$\textit{Amount of gentian violet needed}$$

$$\textit{for } 500 \textit{ ml of } 0.001\% \textit{ solution} =$$

$$\frac{1(mg)}{100,000(ml)} = \frac{x(mg)}{500(ml)}$$

$$x = \frac{1 \times 500}{100,000} = \frac{5}{1000}$$

$$= 0.005 \textit{ mg gentian violet}$$

$$\textit{Amount of gentian violet needed}$$

$$\textit{for 500 ml of 0.003\% solution} =$$

$$\frac{3(mg)}{100,000(ml)} = \frac{x(mg)}{500(ml)}$$

$$x = \frac{3 \times 500}{100,000} = \frac{15}{1000}$$

$$= 0.015 \textit{ mg gentian violet}$$

Example 4. How many grams of pilocarpine nitrate should be used to prepare 25 mL of 2% solution?

$$\frac{2(g)}{100(ml)} = \frac{x(g)}{25(ml)}$$

$$x = \frac{2 \times 25}{100} = \frac{50}{100} = \frac{1}{2}$$

$$= 0.5 \textit{ g pilocarpine nitrate}$$

PRACTICE PROBLEMS

PERCENTAGE AND STRENGTH

1. How many grams of salicylic acid and benzoic acid should be used in preparing 100 grams of an ointment containing 12% and 6% of each, respectively?
2. How many grams of boric acid should be used in compounding the following prescription:

℞

Boric acid	2:100
Aqua add to	90 mL

3. What is the amount of potassium permanganate (in g) that should be used in compounding the following prescription?

℞

Potassium permanganate	0.03%
Aqua ad	600 mL

4. What is the percentage strength of boric acid if 50 grams are dissolved in 350 ml of deionized distilled water?
5. In preparing 500 mL of a topical formulation, a community pharmacist used 8 mL of liquid phenol. What is the percentage strength (v/v) of the liquefied phenol in this topical formulation?
6. In preparation of 100 mL mouthwash, a pharmacist used 250 mg of menthol. What is the percentage (w/v) of menthol in this mouthwash?
7. What is the amount of codeine sulfate to be used in compounding the following prescription?

℞

Codeine sulfate	2%
Aqua add to	150 mL

8. What is the amount of methyl salicylate in (mL) that should be used in compounding the following prescription?

℞

Methyl salicylate	6%
Isopropanol	150 mL

9. What is the amount of peppermint oil (in mL) that should be used in compounding aromatic water in the following prescription?

℞

Peppermint oil	2%
Water to	220 mL

10. How many grams of drug A should be dissolved in 140 mL of distilled water to prepare 8% (w/v) solution?
11. How many grams of a drug substance are needed to prepare 200 mL of a 10% (w/w) solution in water?
12. How many grams of a dorzolamide are needed to prepare 60 mL of a 2% (w/w) ophthalmic solution in isotonic solution?
13. Express each of the following concentrations as a ratio strength:
    a. 2 g of active ingredient in 50 mL of the solution
    b. 0.2 mg of active ingredient in 2 mL of the solution
    c. 25 mg of active ingredient in 5 mL of the solution
    d. 1 mg of active ingredient in 1 mL of the solution
14. How many milligrams of a benzalkonium chloride should be used in preparing 5 liters of a 0.001% solution?
15. A liquid medication contains 2.5 mg of fluoxetine hydrochloride per 75 milliliters. Express the milligram percent (mg%) concentration of this preparation.
16. An injection contains 50 mg pentobarbital sodium in each mL of solution. What is the percentage strength (w/v) of the solution?
17. If 500 g of dextrose monohydrate are dissolved in enough water to make 20 L, what is the percentage strength (w/v) of the solution?
18. How many milliliters of a 0.9% (w/v) of sodium chloride can be prepared from 11.25 g of sodium chloride?
19. If 50 g of magnesium citrate are dissolved in enough water to make 2.5 L, what is the percentage strength (w/v) of the solution?
20. What is the percentage strength (w/w) of a solution made by dissolving 250 g of potassium chloride in 750 mL of water?
21. If 100 mg of docusate sodium are dissolved in water and the volume is made up to 10 mL, what is the percentage strength (w/w) of the solution?
22. A formula for a mouth rinse contains 1/10% (w/v) of zinc chloride. How many grams of zinc chloride should be used in preparing 10 liters of the mouth rinse?
23. What is the percentage strength (w/w) of a solution made by dissolving 0.3 g of cimetidine hydrochloride in 90 g of water?
24. How many milliliters of resorcinol monoacetate liquid should be used to prepare a liter of a 15% (v/v) lotion?
25. How many milligrams of sodium fluoride must be dissolved in 500 mL of water to make 0.05% (w/w) solution?
26. If one liter of a solution contains 250 g of active drug, what is its percentage strength, expressed as w/v?
27. How many grams of calcium carbonate should be used in preparing 100 mL of 10% calcium carbonate suspension?
28. If a patient is instructed to take 250 mL of 16% w/v of an oral solution, how many grams of the drug will he consume?
29. How many grams of iodine are represented in a 20 mL of 20% w/v iodine solution?

30. If 230 mL of a solution contains 46 mg of drug, what is the strength of this solution in percent (w/v)?
31. If 250 mL of a 0.1% solution is mixed with 150 mL of a 0.3% solution, what will be the strength (percent w/v) of the final solution?
32. What is the percent (w/v) strength of a solution that has 500 mg of drug in 200 mL?
33. What is the percentage strength (in w/v) of a 5 mg in 5 mL solution?
34. While preparing 250 mL of 2% (w/v) solution, a pharmacist mistakenly used only 4.5 g of drug. How many more milligrams of this drug are needed to get the correct strength?

ANSWERS

Ratios and Proportions

1. 4:1, 4.0, 400%
2. 1:8, 0.125, 12.5%
3. 1:2, 0.5, 50%
4. 3:1, 3.0, 300%
5. 3:1, 3.0, 300%
6. 40:81, 0.494, 49.38%
7. 0.12 g
8. 1 g of iodine, and 2 g of potassium iodide
9. 20 g
10. Glucose:saline = 1:2
11. 5000 doses
12. 1.2 g
13. 22.5 mg
14. 7.2 mg
15. 30 tablets
16. 10 days
17. 30,000 mg
18. 62.5 g
19. 10 g
20. 1280 mg/10 days
21. 40 mg
22. 0.5 mL
23. 52.4 g
24. 10.2 mg
25. 2.6 mL
26. 240 mg
27. 500 mg
28. 1/100
29. 100 mL
30. 2.5 g
31. 3
32. 750 mg
33. 0.05 mL
34. 4.5 kg
35. 20
36. 50 mL
37. 3
38. 7.5 mL
39. 600
40. 5 mg
41. 550 mg
42. 2 L

Percentage Strength

1. 12 g salicylic acid and 6 g benzoic acid
2. 1.8 g
3. 0.18 g
4. 14.3%
5. 1.6% (v/v)
6. 0.25% (w/v)
7. 3 g
8. 9 mL
9. 4.4 mL

10. 11.2 g
11. 20 g
12. 1.2 g
13. (a) 4%
    (b) 0.01% or 10 mg%
    (c) 0.5% or 500 mg%
    (d) 0.1% or 100 mg%
14. 50 mg
15. 3.3 mg%
16. 5% or 5000 mg%
17. 2.5%
18. 1250 mL
19. 2%
20. 33.33%
21. 1000 mg% or 1 g%
22. 10 g
23. 0.33%
24. 150 mL
25. 250 mg
26. 25%
27. 10 g
28. 40 g
29. 4 g
30. 0.02%
31. 0.175%
32. 0.25%
33. 0.1%
34. 500

4 Applying Systems of Measurements

The knowledge and application of various calculations are essential for the practice of pharmacy and related health professions. Many calculations have been simplified by the shift from apothecary to metric system of measurements. However, a significant proportion of calculation errors occurs because of simple mistakes in arithmetic. Further, the dosage forms prepared by pharmaceutical companies undergo several inspections and quality control tests. Such a system of validation is almost impossible to find in a pharmacy or hospital setting. Therefore it is imperative that the healthcare professionals be extremely careful in performing pharmacy math.

METRIC SYSTEM

The metric system is the most widely used system of measurement in the world. It is federally mandated in the United States and appears in the official listing of drugs in the United States Pharmacopoeia (USP). The metric system of measurement, which was first developed by the French, is a logically organized system and most commonly used for prescribing and administering medications. The basic units, multiplied or divided by 10, make up the metric system, i.e., the units are based on the multiples of ten. Therefore, knowledge of decimals, reviewed in the second chapter, is useful for this system.

In the metric system, the three primary or fundamental units are the meter for length, the liter for volume, and the gram for weight. In addition to these basic units, the metric system includes multiples of basic units with a prefix to indicate their relationship with the basic unit. For example, a milliliter represents 1/1000 or 0.001 part of a liter. A milligram represents 0.001 gram, and a kilogram represents 1000 times the gram. The following tables (Tables 4.1, 4.2 and 4.3) of measurements are very important for the pharmacy and healthcare personnel.

The pharmacist should be able to perform interconversions such as going from a microgram to a gram or from a nanogram to a microgram. The following general guidelines may be helpful:

1. To prevent the problem of overlooking a decimal point, precede the decimal point with a zero if the value is less than one. For example, writing 0.5 g is better than .5 g. As a practical example, if a prescription is written for oxycodone oral solution .5 mg/.5 mL, one possible mistake could be dispensing 0.5 mg/5.0 mL solution. This under-medication to the patient would most likely be avoided if zeros are added and the numbers are expressed as 0.5 mg/0.5 mL.

TABLE 4.1
Metric Weights

	Unit	Abbreviation
One gram (g) is equal to	0.001 kilogram	kg
	0.01 hectogram	hg
	0.1 dekagram	dkg
	10 decigrams	dg
	100 centigrams	cg
	1000 milligrams	mg
	1,000,000 micrograms	µg or mcg
	1,000,000,000 nanograms	ng

TABLE 4.2
Metric Volume

	Unit	Abbreviation
One liter (L) is equal to	0.001 kiloliter	kL
	0.01 hectoliter	hL
	0.1 dekaliter	dkL
	10 deciliters	dL
	100 centiliters	cL
	1000 milliliters	mL
	1,000,000 microliters	µL
	1,000,000,000 nanoliters	nL

TABLE 4.3
Metric Length

	Unit	Abbreviation
One meter (m) is equal to	0.001 kilometer	km
	0.01 hectometer	hm
	0.1 dekameter	dkm
	10 decimeters	dm
	100 centimeters	cm
	1000 millimeters	mm
	1,000,000 micrometers	µm
	1,000,000,000 nanometers	nm

2. To convert a larger unit to a smaller unit (for example, milligram to microgram), multiply by 1,000 or move the decimal point 3 places to the right.
3. To convert a smaller unit to a larger unit (for example, microgram to centigram), divide by 10,000 or simply move the decimal point 4 places to the left.
4. To add, subtract, multiply, or divide different metric units, first convert all the units to the same denomination. For example, to subtract 64 mg from 0.12 g, solve as 120 mg – 64 mg = 56 mg.

   Remember:
   a. Gram is represented by g or G, whereas a grain is represented by gr.
   b. Milliliters are sometimes represented by cc, which is a cubic centimeter (cm^3). This is very useful especially when a conversion from a volume unit to a length unit or vice versa is needed.
   c. Micrograms (μg) can also be represented by mcg.

5. One should be careful with decimal points on prescriptions. When taking a prescription by telephone, decimal points should not be used unless needed. For example, *Norpramine® 10.0 mg* could be mistaken for *Norpramine® 100 mg*. The excess drug may cause adverse reactions such as blurred vision, confusion, flushing, fainting, etc. for the patients.

The above rules can be similarly applied to the conversions of volume and length measurements. The tables for volume (liquid) and length measures are provided in Table 4.2 and Table 4.3. While the weight and volume measurements are the most commonly used, the measure of length is used only in measurements such as the patient's height and body surface area.

Example 1: What is the sum of 0.05 kg and 100.02 g?

Remember:
First convert all the units to the same denomination. Therefore, first convert 0.05 kg into g, or convert 100.02 g into kg and then add them up.

$$0.05\ kg = x\ g$$

$$1\ kg = 1000\ g$$

$$x = \frac{1000 \times 0.05}{1} = \frac{1000 \times 5}{100} = 50\ g$$

So, we can rewrite the problem

using the units of (g) as follows:

$$50\ g + 100.02\ g = 50.00\ g + 100.02\ g = 150.02\ g$$

Example 2. Convert the following metric volumes into their corresponding equivalents:

1. 50 mL into cL
2. 100 hL into L
3. 800 mL into nL

$$\because 1\ L = 1000\ mL = 100\ cL$$

$$\therefore 10\ ml = 1\ cL$$

a. $= 50\ mL = x\ cL$

$$x = \frac{5\theta \times 1}{1\theta} = 5\ cL \qquad \therefore 50\ mL = 5\ cL,\ answer$$

$$\because 0.01\ hL = 1\ L$$

$$\therefore 1\ hL = 100\ L$$

b. $\therefore 100\ hl = x\ L$

$$x\ L = \frac{100 \times 100}{1} = 10{,}000\ L = 1 \times 10^4\ L,\ answer$$

$$\because 1\ L = 1000{,}000{,}000\ nL = 1 \times 10^9\ nL$$

$$\therefore 1\ ml \quad = 10^6\ nL$$

c. $\therefore 800\ mL = x\ nL$

$$x\ nL = \frac{800 \times 10^6}{1} = 8 \times 10^{6+2} = 8 \times 10^8\ nL$$

$$OR \quad 800\ mL = 800{,}000{,}000\ nL,\ answer$$

PRACTICE PROBLEMS

Metric System

1. Add 2 L, 500 cL, and 0.6 hL. Provide the answer in liters.
2. What is the total volume of sodium chloride solution in liters when 500 mL, 0.05 kL, and 10^8 nL of sodium chloride solutions are added together?
3. Add 1.05 g and 200 mg. Provide the answer in mcg.
4. Add 0.55 kg, 55 mg, and 12.5 g. Provide the answer in grams.
5. Add 0.0025 kg, 1750 mg, 2.25 g, and 825,000 mcg. Express the answer in grams.
6. Add 7.25 L and 875 mL. Provide the answer in mL.
7. A sedative liquid medication contains 0.25 mg of an active ingredient per mL. How many mg of the substance will 5 liters contain?

8. Multiply 255 mg by 380, divide the result by 0.85, and reduce the result to grams.
9. If an aspirin tablet contains 75 mg of acetyl salicylic acid per tablet, how many tablets may be prepared from 5.25 kg of aspirin?
10. How many pounds are represented by 250 kg?
11. If a 10-mL ampoule contains 0.125 g of aminophylline, how many mL should be administered to provide a 25-mg dose of aminophylline?
12. An inhalation product provides 240 mg of beclomethasone dipropionate for every 300 inhalations. How many mcg of beclomethasone dipropionate would be contained in each inhalation?
13. Synthroid tablets contain 100 mcg levothyroxine sodium per tablet. How many grams of levothyroxine sodium are needed to make 25,000 tablets?
14. How many tablets, each containing 250 mg of clarithromycin, can be prepared from 5 kg of clarithromycin?
15. An IV solution contains 10 μg of a drug in each mL. How many mg of the drug would a patient receive if a liter of this product is infused?
16. A tablet dosage form indicated for cold contains the following ingredients. How many tablets can be prepared with 0.6 kg of pseudoephedrine (assuming the other ingredients are available in sufficient quantities)?

Acetaminophen	325 mg
Chlorpheniramine Maleate	2 mg
Pseudoephedrine HCl	30 mg
Dextromethorphan HCl	15 mg

17. How many tablets containing 20 mg of dicyclomine HCl can be prepared from 0.8 kg of dicyclomine HCl?
18. Based on the following formula, how many grams of codeine sulfate would be needed to make 200 capsules?

℞

Codeine Sulfate	
Papaverine HCl aa	0.015
Calcium carbonate ad	0.3
Mix to make capsule 1.	

19. A stock solution contained 0.005 kL phosphate buffer. In a series of experiments, 4 L, 2500 μL, and 250 mL were consumed. What is the volume of buffer solutions remaining (in liters) at the end of these experiments?
20. A multivitamin tablet contains 6.15 mg of vitamin B_{12} and twice this amount of vitamin C. How many mg of each vitamin should be used in preparing 500 caplets?
21. How many g of loratidine would be required to make 50,000 tablets, each containing 10 mg of loratidine?
22. How many mg of clonidine would be required to make 25,000 tablets, each containing 0.2 mg of clonidine?
23. An antibiotic liquid preparation contains 50 mg of erythromycin per milliliter. How many mg of erythromycin are contained in 5 liters of this preparation?

24. How many glipizide tablets, each containing 5 mg, can be prepared from 15 g of glipizide?
25. Based on the following formula, how many grams of lactose are needed to prepare 20 capsules?

℞

Phenobarbital		0.540 g
Hyoscine Hydrobromide		4.5 mg
Atropine Sulfate		8.0 mg
Lactose	ad	1.0 g

Mix and prepare 20 hard gelatin capsules.

APOTHECARIES' SYSTEM

Unlike the metric system, which has units for weight, volume, and the length, the apothecaries' system has units for weight and volume only. This is an old system, and its use is rapidly declining. However, some physicians still write prescriptions using this system. A few drug labels that were originally produced under the apothecaries' system still state the apothecaries' equivalent on the label. As a few examples, phenobarbital, aspirin, codeine, sodium bicarbonate, and potassium iodide labels appear in the metric as well as apothecary units.

The basic unit for weight is grain (gr), and that of volume is minim (♏). Unlike the metric units, the amount is expressed in Roman numerals after the apothecaries' symbol. For example, ½ grain is expressed as gr ss and not ½ gr. Twenty minims are expressed as ♏-xx. Sometimes some physicians also use Arabic numerals in the apothecary system. For example, 12 ounces can be written as ℥-XII or 12-oz and 4 ounces as ℥-IV or 4-oz. Tables 4.4 and 4.5 show the relationships between measures of liquid volume and solid weight in the apothecaries' system.

TABLE 4.4
Apothecaries' Liquid Measures

60 minims (♏)	=	1 fluid dram (fʒ)
8 fluid drams (fʒ)	=	1 fluid ounce (f℥)
16 fluid ounces (f℥)	=	1 pint (pt or O)
2 pints (O)	=	1 quart (qt)
4 quarts (qt)	=	1 gallon (gal or C)

TABLE 4.5
Apothecaries' Weight Measures

20 grains (gr)	=	1 scruple (℈)
3 scruples (℈)	=	1 dram (ʒ)
8 drams (ʒ)	=	1 ounce (℥)
12 ounces (℥)	=	1 pound (lb)
1 pound (lb)	=	5760 grains (gr)

Example 1:

If a prescription calls for gr iii thyroid desiccated tablets and the pharmacist has gr ss tablets in stock, how many tablets of gr ss should be provided?

gr iii = 3 grains
gr ss = ½ grain
3/½ = 6 tablets of gr ss, answer

Example 2:

How many doses of f℥ iv are present in O ii of Maalox®?

O ii = 2 pints
= 2×16 ounces = 32 ounces
= $32 \times 8 = 256$ fluid drams
= 256/4 = 64 doses, answer

Example 3:

A doctor ordered morphine sulfate gr 3/5, and the pharmacist has a stock solution of gr 1/8 per mL of morphine sulfate. How many mL of the stock solution is required to fill the prescription?

gr 3/5 = 0.6 grains needed
gr 1/8 = 0.125 grains per mL
0.125/mL = 0.6/X
X = 0.6/0.125
or X = 4.8 mL of the stock solution, answer

PRACTICE PROBLEMS

Apothecaries' System

1. If two quarts of generic Tylenol elixir are present in the inventory, how many f℥-iv prescriptions can be filled?
2. If approximately 12 prescriptions of f℥-vi Ventolin® syrup are filled per day, how many gallons of the syrup would be used in 15 days?
3. How many minims of a topical keratolytic solution are contained in a 4-fluid-dram bottle?
4. If 36 APAP suppositories of 2 grains each are dispensed, how many scruples of drug are dispensed?
5. How many apothecary ounces are represented in lbs iiiss?
6. How many fluid drams remain after 4 fluid drams, 60 minims, and 1/2 fluid ounce of Robitussin (generic) are removed from one pint of a solution?
7. How many ounces are represented in gr CXX?
8. A prescription requires gr 1/200 of a drug. If a pharmacist has gr 1/100 scored-tablets, how many tablets should be dispensed?

9. If a generic syrup costs $14 for ½ oz (apoth) and the brand syrup costs $32 for the same amount of syrup, what is the difference in price (in dollars) for one gallon of the drug?
10. The container for Seconal® sodium capsules shows a strength of 100 mg (1½ gr) of the drug secobarbital sodium. If an ounce of drug is available, how many capsules can be prepared?
11. If 4 quarts syrup are available, how many 5 fluid ounce prescriptions can be filled?
12. If 4 pints of solutions are to be dispensed from 10 quarts of stock, how many f℥ will remain in the stock?
13. How many 5 fluid ounce prescriptions can be filled from 30 quarts of a stock solution?
14. How many 8 fluid dram prescriptions can be filled from 3 quarts of solution?
15. If 10 prescriptions of Tylenol elixir containing 80 minims each are to be dispensed per day, how many pints of Tylenol elixir will be used in 30 days?
16. If 100 prescriptions of a topical solution containing 16 minims each are to be dispensed per day, how many quarts of solution will be used in 40 days?
17. If 21 prescriptions of a topical solution containing 50 f℥ each are to be dispensed in a day, how many gallons of solution will be used in 20 days?
18. In order to dispense 15 prescriptions of Tylenol elixir, each containing 12 fluid ounces, how many gallons of Tylenol elixir solution will be used?
19. How many fluid drams of a topical solution are represented in 8 gallons of solution?
20. How many f℥ of a topical solution are contained in a 24-gallon stock solution?
21. How many pints of a topical solution are in a 40 gallon bottle?
22. How many minims of a topical solution are represented in 28 pints of solution?
23. If 20 tablets, each containing 4 drams of a drug are dispensed, how many ounces of drug are dispensed?
24. If 57 capsules, each containing 5 scruples, are dispensed, how many ounces of drug are dispensed in total?
25. If 26 capsules of 4 drams each are dispensed, how many ounces of drug are dispensed?
26. If 324 tablets of 3 grains each are dispensed, how many pounds of drug are dispensed?
27. How many apothecary scruples are represented in ℥-xss?
28. How many apothecary drams are represented in lbs-xxii?
29. How many apothecary grains are represented in ℥-xiiss?
30. How many apothecary drams are present in lbs-cx?
31. How many scruples remain after withdrawing 20 scruples, 60 grains, and 2 drams from a 1-lb container?
32. How many f℥ remain after removing 16 f℥, 14 f℥, and 2 pints Robitussin from a 1-gallon container?

33. How many minims remain after removing 5 fʒ, 120 ♏, and 0.5 fʒ Robitussin from a 1 f℥ container?
34. How many fʒ remain after withdrawing 5 fʒ, 180 ♏, and 1 f℥ Robitussin from a 1 pint container?
35. How many grains are represented in lb XX?
36. How many ʒ are represented in lbs-vii?
37. How many ℥ are represented in gr-civ?
38. How many ʒ are contained in gr-cxx?
39. A prescription requires gr-ii drug, and the pharmacist has gr-ss scored tablets. How many tablets should be dispensed?
40. A prescription requires gr-iv drugs, and the pharmacist has gr-ii scored tablets. How many tablets should be dispensed?
41. A prescription requires gr-xii drugs, and the pharmacist has gr-ss scored tablets. How many tablets should be dispensed?
42. A prescription requires ℈-iiss drug, and the pharmacist has gr-v scored tablets. How many tablets should be dispensed?
43. If a generic syrup costs $12 for ½ oz and the brand syrup costs $16 for ½ oz, what is the difference in price per gallon?
44. If a generic syrup costs $24 for ½ oz and the brand syrup costs $58 for the same quantity, what is the difference in price per pint?
45. If a generic syrup costs $18 for 1 oz and the brand syrup costs $36 for the same amount, what is the difference in price per gallon?
46. If a generic syrup costs $37 for 1 pint and the brand syrup costs $45 for the same, what is the price difference per gallon?
47. Seconal sodium capsules are prepared at a strength of 2 grains of secobarbital sodium per capsule. If 1 lb of secobarbital sodium is available, how many capsules can be prepared?
48. According to the label on a container of Seconal sodium capsules, each capsule contains 6 drams of drug secobarbital sodium. If 1 lb of secobarbital sodium is available, how many capsules can be prepared from it?
49. A container for Seconal sodium capsules shows a strength of 6 grains of secobarbital sodium per capsule. If 2 oz of secobarbital sodium are available, how many capsules can be prepared from it?
50. A container for Seconal sodium capsules shows a strength of 2 scruples of secobarbital sodium per capsule. If 1 oz of secobarbital sodium is available, how many capsules can be prepared from it?

HOUSEHOLD CONVERSIONS

Though inaccurate, the household system of measurements is on the rise because of increased home healthcare delivery. In this system, patients use household measuring devices such as the teaspoon, dessertspoon, tablespoon, wineglass, and coffee cup, among others.

In the past, a drop has been used as an equivalent of a minim. However, such a measure should be discouraged because of many factors affecting the drop size, which include the density of the medication, temperature, surface tension, diameter and opening of the dropper, and the angle of the dropper. The official medicinal dropper, according to the United States Pharmacopoeia-National Formulary (USP-NF) delivers 20 drops per mL of water at 25° C. Some manufacturers provide specially calibrated droppers with their products. A few examples of medications containing droppers include Tylenol® pediatric drops, Advil® pediatric drops, and Neosynephrine® nasal drops. Several ear, nose, and eye medications are now available in calibrated containers, which provide drops by gently pressing the containers. Sometimes, the healthcare professional has to calibrate the dropper for measuring small quantities such as 0.1 mL or 0.15 mL, when the manufacturer does not supply the calibrated dropper. The calibration procedure is as follows:

Calibration of the Medicinal Dropper

A dropper is calibrated by counting the number of drops required to transfer 2-mL of the intended liquid from its original container to a 5-mL measuring cylinder. For example, if it takes 40 drops to measure 2 mL of a liquid, then the number of drops to measure 0.15 mL of the liquid is obtained by the method of proportion as follows:

$$\frac{2(mL)}{40(drops)} = \frac{0.15(mL)}{X(drops)}$$

$$X = \frac{0.15 \times 40}{2} = 3$$

$$= 3 drops, answer$$

It is important to remember that the household system of measurement should not be used for calculations in compounding or conversions from one system to the other. The household system of measurement is designed for the convenience to the patient. Therefore this system is used for the directions on labels for the patients. Some common household measures are shown in the following table (Table 4.6).

Interconversions

In many clinical situations, healthcare professionals encounter more than one system of measurement. Therefore, it becomes necessary to convert all quantities to the same system of measurement. Depending upon the circumstances and the degree of accuracy required, a particular system would be preferred over the others. Some commonly used equivalents in pharmacy practice are shown in Table 4.7 and Table 4.8.

A pharmacy or healthcare institution may use a particular set of equivalents as their established standards for their interconversions. The healthcare professionals working in their environment must use that standard. If such standards are not established, generally, the equivalents shown in the right column of Table 4.6 may be used.

TABLE 4.6
Household Measures

Unit	Abbreviation or Symbol	Equivalent Volume in Milliliters
1 teaspoonful	tsp or t	5 mL
1 dessertspoonful	dssp	8 mL
1 tablespoonful	tbsp, T	15 mL
1 ounce	℥	2 tbsp; 30 mL
1 wine-glass	—	30 mL
1 coffee cup	—	6 fluid ounces (f℥ vi); 180 mL
1 glass	—	8 fluid ounces (f℥ viii); 240 mL
1 quart	qt	1000 mL
1 gallon	gal, C	4000 mL

TABLE 4.7
Conversion Equivalents of the Measurement Systems

Apothecary	Metric (precise)	Household (approximate)
1minim (♏)	0.06 mL	—
16.23 minims (♏)	1 mL	—
1 fluid dram (fʒ)	3.69 mL	1 teaspoonful or 5 mL
½ fluid ounce (f℥)	15 mL	1 tablespoonful (tbsp)
1 fluid ounce (f℥)	30 mL	2 tablespoonfuls (tbsp)
1 pint (pt, O)	473 mL	500 mL
1 quart (qt)	946 mL	1 liter

Note. ss = ½

Examples: For the following values, write the precise interpretation either in milliliters (mL) or milligrams (mg).

1. 5 ♏
2. 2.5 f℥
3. fʒ xii
4. f℥ viss
5. 2 tbsp
6. 2 tsp
7. gr $\frac{1}{4}$
8. qt vii
9. pt iss
10. XII gal

TABLE 4.8
Approximate Equivalents Used by Health Professionals

Apothecary	Metric	Commonly Used Equivalent
1 grain (gr)	64.8 mg	65 mg[a]
1 ounce (℥)	31.1 g	30 g
1 pound	373.2 g	454 g[b]
1 minim (♏)	0.062 mL	0.06 mL
1 fluid ounce (f℥)	29.57 mL	30 mL
128 (f℥)	3785 mL	1 gallon (G)
1 Kg	2.2 lbs	

[a] It should be remembered that this conversion is only approximate. Several other approximations have been used on the labels of certain tablets. For example, Saccharin tablets from Eli Lilly Co. show ½ gr (32 mg) on their label, whereas the phenobarbital tablets from the same company have 30 mg (½ gr) on their label. Similarly, sodium bicarbonate tablets from Eli Lilly have 5 gr (325 mg) on their label, and potassium iodide from the same company has 300 mg (5 gr) on its container label. In this book, it is recommended to use one grain (gr) equivalent to 65 mg.

[b] This amount represents the equivalent of 1 avoirdupois pound. Since the pound is a bulk quantity, use of the avoirdupois system of measurements unit is more common.

Answers:

1. 5 ♏
   1 minim = 0.06 mL
   5 minims = 5 × 0.06 = 0.3 mL, *answer*
2. 2.5 f℥
   1 fluid ounce = 30 mL
   2.5 fluid ounces = 2.5 × 30 = 75 mL, *answer*
3. fʒ xii
   1 fluid dram = 3.69 mL
   12 luid drams = 12 × 3.69 = 44.28 or 44 mL, *answer*
4. f℥ viss
   1 fluid ounce = 30 mL
   6.5 fluid ounces = 6.5 × 30 = 195 mL, *answer*
5. 3 tbsp
   1 tablespoonful = 15 mL
   3 tablespoonfuls = 3 × 15 = 45 mL, *answer*
6. 2 tsp
   1 teaspoonful = 5 mL
   2 teaspoonfuls = 5 × 2 = 10 mL, *answer*

7. $gr\frac{1}{4}$
   1 grain = 65 mg
   ¼ grain = ¼ × 65 = 16.25 mg, *answer*
8. qt vii
   1 quart = 946 mL
   7 quarts = 946 × 7 = 6622 mL, *answer*
9. pt iss
   1 pint = 473 mL
   1.5 pints = 473 × 1.5 = 709.5 or 710 mL, *answer*
10. xii gal
    1 gallon = 3785 mL
    12 gallons = 12 × 3785 = 45,420 mL, *answer*

PRACTICE PROBLEMS

Household Conversions

1. How many fluid ounces fill the volume of 5 coffee cups?
2. How many glasses are contained in 40 fluid ounces?
3. How many tablespoons are contained in 17 ounces?
4. 120 cc is how many tablespoons?
5. How many teaspoons are contained in 1 glass solution?
6. How many wine glasses can be filled from two quarts of a solution?
7. How many tablespoons are contained in 10 fluid ounces?
8. How many tablespoons can be administered from a bottle containing 90 mL?
9. 60 teaspoonfuls are how many fluid ounces?
10. How many coffee cups (approximately) can be filled from 3.6 quarts?
11. 500 mg of tetracycline syrup is ordered; available solution contains 125 mg/teaspoon. How many teaspoons are administered?
12. A medication order calls for Lasix 20 mg by intravenous administration; available solution contains 10 mg/cc. How many milliliters are administered?
13. If a hair shampoo costs $5.6 per 10 f℥, how many mL can be purchased with $35?
14. How many 2 ounce bottles (approximately) can be filled from 3 gallons of an aftershave lotion?
15. 30 mg of Demerol is ordered; available solution contains 500 mcg/cc. How many tablespoons can be given?
16. If a prescription is required for Phenergan VC syrup with codeine, 2 teaspoonfuls at bedtime for 12 days, how many fluid ounces of the syrup would the pharmacist dispense?
17. How many mg of amoxacilline trihydrate are needed to prepare 550 ♍ oral suspension if each mL contain 25 mg of the drug?
18. A pharmacist had a gallon of 2% boric acid lotion; in a series of sales operations, he sold 300 ♍, f℥ v, f℥ xss, and q tiii. What volume, in fluid ounces, of the lotion was left?

19. How many milligrams of dexamethasone are needed to formulate 100 tablets, each tablet containing 1/5 gr of dexamethasone?
20. How many f℥ v bottles can be prepared from 50 gallons of a dermatological lotion?
21. Mr. Adams has been advised to take at least 1.2 liters of an electrolyte solution per day. How many glassfuls should he take in a day?
22. Mrs. Winters takes 1½ (iss) gr phenobarbital sodium tablet twice a day. What is the total amount of (in milligrams) of phenobarbital sodium would she take in 4 days?
23. How many milligrams of brinzolamide should be used to prepare 2% ophthalmic drops of isotonic brinzolamide solution?

℞

Brinzolamide	?
Isotonic solution	f℥ ii

24. How many fluid ounces of the isotonic solution should be used to prepare 0.65% ophthalmic drops of timolol with the amount prescribed below?

℞

Timolol	gr xxx
Isotonic solution	?

25. How many mg of each ingredient should be used to prepare the following medication order?

℞

Codeine phosphate	gr iii
Acetaminophen	gr vii
Caffeine	gr ss

ANSWERS

Metric System

1. 67 L
2. 50.6 L
3. 1.25×10^6 mg
4. 562.56 g
5. 7.33 g
6. 8125 ml
7. 1250 mL
8. 114.0 g
9. 7×10^4
10. 2.5 10^5 g, 550 lb
11. 2 mL
12. 800 μg
13. 25 g
14. 2×10^4 tablets
15. 10 mg
16. 2×10^4 tablets
17. 4×10^4 tablets
18. 3 g
19. 747.5 mL
20. 3075 mg of vitamin B_{12} and 6150 mg of vitamin C
21. 500 g

22. 5000 mg
23. 2.5×10^5 mg
24. 3000 tablets
25. 8.95 g

Apothecaries' System

1. 16 prescriptions
2. 8.44 gallons
3. 240 minims
4. 3.6 scruples
5. 42 ounces
6. 119 fluid drams
7. 0.25 or ¼ ounce
8. 0.5 or ½ tablet
9. $4608
10. 320 capsules
11. 25.6 or 25 prescriptions
12. 256 fluid ounces
13. 192 prescriptions
14. 96 fluid drams
15. 3.125 pints
16. 4.17 quarts
17. 164 gallons
18. 1.40 gallons
19. 8192 fluid drams
20. 3072 fluid ounces
21. 320 pints
22. 215040 minims
23. 1.33 drams
24. 11.9 ounces
25. 13 ounces
26. 0.17 pounds
27. 252 scruples
28. 2112 drams
29. 750 grains
30. 10560 drams
31. 259 scruples
32. 80 fluid ounces
33. 30 minims
34. 112 fluid drams
35. 115200 grains
36. 672 drams
37. 0.22 ounces
38. 2 drams
39. 4 tablets
40. 2 tablets
41. 24 tablets
42. 10 tablets
43. $1024
44. $1088
45. $2304
46. $64
47. 2880 capsules
48. 16 capsules
49. 160 capsules
50. 12 capsules

Household Conversions

1. 30 f℥
2. 5 glasses
3. 34 tbsp
4. 8 tbsp
5. 48 tsp
6. 66 wine glasses
7. 20 tbsp
8. 6 tbsp
9. 10 f℥
10. 20 coffee cups
11. 4 tsp
12. 2 mL
13. 1875 mL
14. 200 bottles
15. 4 tbsp
16. 4 f℥
17. 825 mg
18. 464 mL
19. 1300 mg
20. 1261
21. 5
22. 780 mg
23. 1200 mg
24. 10 f℥
25. Codeine phosphate = 195 mg; acetaminophen = 455 mg; caffeine = 32.5 mg

5 Interpreting Medication Orders

The interpretation of prescription medication orders is one of the most important requirements of pharmacy practice. According to the National Association of Boards of Pharmacy's (NABP's) Model State Pharmacy Act, "The 'Practice of Pharmacy' shall mean the interpretation and evaluation of prescription orders; the compounding, dispensing, labeling of drugs and devices (except labeling by a manufacturer, packer, or distributor of non-prescription drugs and commercially packaged legend drugs and devices); the participation in drug selection and drug utilization reviews; the proper and safe storage of drugs and devices and the maintenance of proper records, therefore; the responsibility of advising where necessary or where regulated, of therapeutic values, content, hazards and use of drugs and devices; and the offering or performing of those acts, services, operations or transactions necessary in the conduct, operation, management and control of pharmacy."

The Model State Pharmacy Act of the NABP also defines drugs that are to be dispensed with or without prescription. "'Prescription Drug or Legend Drug' shall mean a drug which, under Federal Law is required, prior to being dispensed or delivered, to be labeled with either of the following statements: (1) 'Caution: Federal law prohibits dispensing without prescription' (2) 'Caution: Federal and State law restricts this drug to use by or on the order of a licensed veterinarian'; or a drug which is required by any applicable Federal or State Law or regulation to be dispensed on prescription only or is restricted to use by practitioners only." Non-prescription drugs are defined as "Non-narcotic medicines or drugs which may be sold without a prescription and which are prepackaged for use by the consumer and labeled in accordance with the requirements of the statutes and regulation of this State and the Federal Government."

The definitions provided above underscore the importance of understanding and interpreting prescriptions. A prescription is defined as an order for medication from a doctor, dentist, veterinarian, or any other licensed healthcare professional authorized to prescribe in that state. It shows the relationship between the prescriber, patient, and the pharmacist, in which the latter provides the medication to the patient.

TYPES OF PRESCRIPTIONS

Pharmacists receive prescriptions by telephone, fax, as written prescriptions from individual doctors, doctors practicing in a group, or hospitals and other institutions. Telephone orders are reduced to a written prescription (hard copy) by pharmacists. Generally prescriptions include printed forms called "prescription blanks" which include the name, address, and telephone number of the prescribing physician; a provision to write the name, address, age and date of birth of the patient; and the ℞ symbol. "Medication orders" are prescription equivalents, which are written by physicians in a hospital or similar institutions. Components of medication orders with appropriate examples are presented in the next section.

PARTS OF A PRESCRIPTION

Generally, prescriptions consist of the following parts:

1. Prescriber's name, degree, address and telephone number. In the case of prescriptions coming from a hospital or a multi-center clinic, the hospital or clinic's name, address and telephone numbers appear at the top. In such a case, the physician's name and degree would appear near his/her signature.
2. Patient's name, address, age, and the date of prescription.
3. The *superscription*, which is represented by the Latin sign, ℞. This sign represents "take thou" or "you take" or "recipe." Sometimes, this sign is also used for the pharmacy itself.
4. The *inscription* is the general content of the prescription. It states the name and quantity of the medication, either as its brand (proprietary) or generic (nonproprietary) names. In the case of compounded prescriptions, the *inscription* states the name and quantity of active ingredients.
5. The *subscription* represents the directions to the dispenser and indicates the type of dosage form or the number of dosage units. For compounded prescriptions, the subscription is written using English or Latin abbreviations (Table 5.1 through Table 5.7). A few examples are provided as follows:
   a. M. et ft. sol. Disp ℥ ix (Mix and make solution. Dispense nine fluidounces)
   b. Ft. ung. Disp ℥ iv (Make ointment and dispense four ounces)
   c. Ft. cap. DTD xii (Make capsules and let 12 such doses be given)
6. The *signa*, also known as *transcription,* represents the directions to the patient. These directions are written in English or Latin or a combination of both (Table 5.1 through Table 5.7). Latin directions in prescriptions are declining, but since they are still used, it is important to learn them. A few examples are provided below:
   a. ii caps tid, 7 days (Take two capsules thrice daily for seven days)
   b. gtt. iii a.u. hs (Instill three drops in both the ears at bed time)
   c. In rect. prn pain (Insert rectally as needed for pain)
7. The prescriber's signature.
8. The refill directions, in which the information about how many times (if authorized) a prescription can be refilled, are provided.
9. Other information, such as "Dispense as Written."
10. Drug Enforcement Administration (DEA) registration number and/or the state registration number of the prescribing authority.

Dr. John Doe
4301 E Markham St, Little Rock, AR 76543
Phone No. 501-555-1000

Name: Brittany Taylor **Age:** 72
Address: 95 Chenal Blvd, Hope **Date:** 5/28/03
Pχ
Darvocet-N 100
#30
Sig: bid, prn pain.

Refills none
DAW √
Dr. John Doe
DEA #AI7973142

FIGURE 5.1 Sample prescription.

CHENAL PHARMACY
169 Hillside Avenue
Little Rock, AR 71206 555-0342

Pχ # 123456 Date: 5/28/03
Taylor, Brittany
95 Chenal Blvd.

Take one tablet twice daily, as needed for pain.
Darvocet-N 100 tablets, #30
John Doe, M.D.

FIGURE 5.2 Matching label.

SAMPLE PRESCRIPTION

Label Requirements

It is a legal requirement to affix a prescription label (Figure 5.1) on the immediate container of prescription medications. The pharmacist is responsible for the accuracy of the label. It should bear the name, address, and the telephone number of the pharmacy, the date of dispensing, the prescription number, the prescriber's name, the name and address of the patient, and the directions for use of the medication. Some states also require additional information. The name and strength of the medication and the refill directions are also written frequently. The label for the sample prescription is shown in Figure 5.2.

MEDICATION ORDER

While prescriptions are written in an outpatient setting, physicians in a hospital setting write medication orders. A medication order is also known as a drug order or a physician's order. These orders generally contain the name, address of the patient, age or date of birth, hospital ID number, room number, the date of admission into the hospital, and any patient allergies. Sometimes the patient's diagnosis is included. Besides patient information, the following information about the medication is included.

- Date and time of the medication order
- Name of the drug (brand or generic)
- Dosage form
- Route of administration, e.g., oral, intramuscular, intravenous, etc.

- Administration schedule, e.g., times per day, milliliters per hour, at bedtime, etc.
- Other information such as some restrictions or specifications.
- Physician's signature
- Provision for the pharmacist's or nurses' notes

HILLTON HEALTH CARE HOSPITAL **LITTLE ROCK, ARKANSAS**				
PHYSICIAN'S ORDER SHEET			Goldman, Brown 41-22 Passedena Little Rock, AK ID# 87654	Admit 2/26/96 DOB 7/7/42 Dr. L. Bailey Room 107
Please Use Ball Point Pen and Press Firmly. You are making more than one copy				
ORDERED		**PHYSICIAN'S ORDERS** START A NEW SECTION WITH EACH SET OF ORDERS	NURSE NOTED	
DATE	TIME		HOUR	NAME
2/26	0900	Dynapen 250 mg. PO q6h		
2/26	0900	Darvon Compound 65 PO q4h prn pain		
2/26	0900	Vibramycin 0.2 g po stat	0940	L. Ito
		L. Bailey, M.D.		

FIGURE 5.3 Sample medication order.

COMMON LATIN TERMS AND ABBREVIATIONS

TABLE 5.1
Terms Related to Quantities

Abbreviation	Term/Phrase	Meaning
aa	ana	of each
q.s., q.s.	quantum sufficiat	sufficient quantity
ad lib.	ad libitum	freely, at pleasure
℥	ounce	one ounce
f℥	fluid ounce	one fluid ounce
O or pt	pint	one pint
qt	quart	one quart
gal	gallon	one gallon
♏	minim	one minim
ʒ	dram or drachm	one drachm
fʒ	fluid drachm	one fluid drachm
gr	grain	one grain
℈	scruple	one scruple

TABLE 5.2
Terms Related to Administration Times/Dosage Frequency

Abbreviation	Term/Phrase	Meaning
qd or q.d.	quaque die	once daily
bid or b.i.d.	bis in die	twice daily
tid or t.i.d.	ter in die	three times daily
qid or q.i.d.	quarter in die	four times daily
am or AM	ante meridium	in the morning
pm or PM	post meridium	in the evening
h.s.	hora somni	at bed time
a.c.	ante cibos	before meals
p.c.	post cibos	after meals
i.c.	inter cibos	between meals
om	omne mane	every morning
on	omne nocte	every night
p.r.n.	pro re nata	when necessary
q.h.	quaque hora	every hour
q2h	quaque secunda hora	every two hours
q3h	quaque tertia hora	every three hours
q4h	quaque quarta hora	every four hours
q6h	quaque sex hora	every six hours
q8h	quaque octo hora	every eight hours

TABLE 5.3
Terms Related to Formulations or Products

Abbreviation	Term/Phrase	Meaning
amp	ampul	ampul
aur or oto	auristillae	ear drops
cap	Capsula	a capsule
comp	compositus	compounded
cm or crem	cremor	a cream
garg	gargarisma	gargle
gtt	guttae	drops
inj.	injectio	an injection
liq.	liquor	a solution
mist.	mistura	a mixture
Neb.	nebula	a nebulizer
pil.	pilula	a pill
pulv.	pulvis	a powder
suppos.	suppositorium	a suppository
troch.	trochiscus	a lozenge
tab	tablet	a tablet

TABLE 5.4
Instructions for Preparations

Abbreviation	Term/Phrase	Meaning
div.	divide	divide
ft	fiat	let it be made
m. ft.	misce fiat	mix to make
d.t.d.	dentur tales doses	such doses be given
e.m.p.	ex modo prescriptio	in the manner prescribed
s, s̄	sine	without
c, c̄	cum	with

TABLE 5.5
Method of Application

Abbreviation	Term/Phrase	Meaning
o.d. or OD	oculus dexter	right eye
o.l. or OL	oculus Lævus	left eye
o.u. or O_2	oculo utro	each eye or both eyes
o.s. or OS	oculo sinister	left eye
a.d. or AD	aurio dextra	right ear
a.l. or AL	aurio Læva	left ear
e.m.p.	ex. modo prescriptio	as directed
u.d.	ut. dictum	as directed
c, Ê	cum	with
dext	dexter	right
s, ú	sine	without
s	sinister	left

TABLE 5.6
Vehicles/IV Solutions

Abbreviation	Meaning
aq	water
aq. bull	boiling water
DW/or aq. Dist	distilled water
D5W	dextrose 5% in water
NS	normal saline (0.9% sodium chloride)
½NS	half strength of normal saline
RL	ringer's lactate
LR	lactated Ringer's

TABLE 5.7
Miscellaneous Abbreviations

Abbrev.	Meaning	Abbreviation	Meaning
AUD	apply as directed	IVPB	intravenous piggybag
ASA	acetyl salicylic acid	min	minutes
APAP	acetaminophen	MVI	multivitamin infusion
BCP	birth control pills	MOM	milk of Magnesia
BIW	twice a week	N & V	nausea and vomiting
BM	bowel movement	NPO	nothing by mouth
BP	blood pressure	NR	non repeatable or No refill
BS	blood sugar	NTG	nitroglycerin
BSA	body surface area	p.o.	per oral, by mouth
CHF	congestive heart failure	PBZ	pyribenzamine
DSS	doccusate	PPA	phenylpropanolamine
EES	erythromycin ethyl succinate	QOD	every other day
et	and	SOB	shortness of breadth
fl	fluid	SC	subcutaneous
FA	folic acid	SL	sublingual
HA	head ache	ss	one-half
HC	hydrocortisone	stat	immediately, at once
HCTZ	hydrochlorothiazide	tal. dos	such doses
HT	hypertension	tsp, t	teaspoon
ID	intradermal	tbsp, T	tablespoon
IM	intramuscular	TIW	thrice a week
INH	isoniazid	TPN	total parenteral nutrition
IOP	intraocular pressure	URI	upper respiratory infection
IV	intravenous	UTI	urinary tract infection

EXAMPLES

Interpret the following medication orders:

1. Cortisporin Otic gtts ii a.u. tid et h.s.
   Interpretation. Administer 2 drops of cortisporin otic in both ears 3 times a day and at bedtime.
2. Tetracycline 500 mg p.o. q.d.
   Interpretation. Give 500 mg of tetracycline orally once a day.
3. Morphine sulfate gr ½ IM q4 p.r.n., pain
   Interpretation. Administer ½ grain of morphine sulfate intramuscularly every 4 hours as needed for pain

Solve the following:

1. How many f℥ of amoxicillin suspension would the patient receive?

 ℞

 Amoxicillin 125 mg/5 mL
 Sig: ii tsp tid, 7 days
 Solution:
 2×5 mL = 10 mL, each dose
 $10 \times 3 = 30$ mL per day
 $30 \times 7 = 210$ mL or f℥ vii for 7 days, answer.

2. If the pharmacist has only 250 mg capsules in the inventory, how many capsules should be given to the patient?

 ℞

 Keflex caps 500 mg
 Sig: i cap bid, 10 days
 Solution: Four 250 mg capsules per day and therefore 40 capsules for 10 days.

3. How many grams of aspirin are needed for the following prescription?

 ℞

 Aspirin gr iv
 Caffeine gr iss
 Ft. cap. DTD #XXV
 Solution: Each capsule contains 4 grains = $65 \times 4 = 260$ mg; for 25 capsules, the amount of aspirin needed is = $260 \times 25 = 6500$ mg or 6.5 g, answer.

PRACTICE PROBLEMS

Interpret the following medication orders:

1. Atrovent® Inhaler (ipratoprium bromide): ii inhalations qid, ud
2. Betoptic® (betaxolol HCl): ii gtt, ou bid, ud
3. Blocadren® 10 mg (timolol maleate): i tab qd, prn migraine
4. Capoten® 50 mg (captopril): ss tab stat, i tid, ud
5. Cartrol® 5 mg (carteolol HCl): i tab stat, ii qd
6. Catapress TTS®-2 Patch (clonidine HCl): Apply to upper arm or chest, q7d, ud
7. Clinoril® 200 mg (sulindac): i tab bid, pc, 10 days
8. Doxycycline 100 mg (Vibramycin®): i cap bid, 10 days
9. Duricef® 1g (cefadroxil monohydrate): i qd, 10 days
10. Diflucan® 100 mg (fluconazole): ii stat, i qd

11. Diphenhydramine HCl Syrup (Benadryl®): i tsp tid, and ii tsp hs
12. E-Mycin® 333 mg (erythromycin): i q8h, p.c., 7 days
13. Fiorinal[7]® (aspirin, butalbital, caffeine): ii caps, q4h prn, pain
14. Habitrol® 14 mg (nicotine TDDS): i patch qd, 8 wks
15. K-Lor® oral solution (potassium chloride): M i tsp in glassful of OJ and drink
16. Lomotil® (diphenoxylate HCl+atropine sulfate): i tsp tid, prn diarrhea
17. Maxair® Autohaler (pirbuterol acetate): ii puffs q4–6h, UD
18. Normodyne® 200 mg (labetolol HCl): i tab bid, ic
19. Pediazole® susp (erythromycin es+sulfisoxazole acetyl): i tsp q6h, 10 days
20. Prednisone 5 mg (Deltasone,® Orasone®): ii tab tid, ud
21. Reglan® 5 mg (metoclopramide HCl): i tab bid, ac and i hs
22. Suprax® 200 mg (cefixime): i bid, finish all
23. Terazol® 7 cm (terconazole): i applicatorful in vag, qhs, 7 days
24. Tobrex® op oint (tobramycin): ½ inch, bid-tid, in affected eye, UD
25. Toradol® 10 mg tab (ketorolac tromethamine): i po, qid × 5 days, UD
26. If a medication order reads "Insulin 200 units/cc, # 10 cc; Sig: 10 units bid, sc," how many days would the medication last?
27. If the available atropine vial reads gr 1/150 per mL, how many milliliters of the injection should be administered?

    ℞

    Atropine Sulfate 0.3 mg
    Sig: Administer intramuscularly

28. How many grams of aspirin would be needed to fill the following prescription?

    ℞

    Aspirin gr v
    Caffeine gr i
    Lactose qs
    Ft. cap. DTD # xx

29. If a calibrated dropper delivers 40 drops per 2-mL, how many drops should the patient instill in each ear every time?

    ℞

    Dr. Zogg's otic drops 15 cc
    Sig: 0.1 cc au tid, prn

30. How many grams of acetaminophen are needed to compound the following prescription?

    ℞

    Acetaminophen gr xx
    Codeine phosphate gr v
    M. et. Ft. cap. # xx
    Sig. i q 8 hr prn pain

31. How many milligrams of codeine phosphate are required to compound the following prescription?

    ℞

    Codeine phosphate gr viiss
    Lactose q.s. gr C
    M. et. Ft. DTD cap. # xx
    Sig. 1 q 6 hr, prn pain

32. If the available atropine vial reads gr 1/110 per mL, how many milliliters of the injection should be administered?

    ℞

    Atropine Sulfate 0.6 mg
    Sig: Administer intramuscularly

33. If a medication order reads "Inderal 20 mg p.o. t.i.d." and the pharmacy has 10 mg tablets of inderal, how many tablets can be given for a 3- day supply?
34. If a medication order reads "Duricef 1 g p.o. qid ac for 10 days" and if 500 mg tablets are in stock, how many tablets are dispensed?
35. When a prescription for Tylenol with codeine was called in as, "gr i p.o. q4h p.r.n. pain," and the supply has tylenol with codeine 30 mg, 65 mg and 100 mg tablets, which of these tablets may be dispensed?
36. If a medication order reads, "Motrin 600 mg p.o., b.i.d.," and the patient has 32 capsules 300 mg/each, how many days would his supply last?
37. If a medication order reads, "Lanoxin 0.25 mg, p.o., q.d.," how many 0.125 mg tablets of lanoxin should be dispensed to last the patient for 10 days?
38. How many fluid ounces of Dimetapp elixir are needed to fill the following prescription?

    ℞

    Benadryl elixir
    Dimetapp elixir aa q.s. 120 mL

39. If a physician order reads "Trandate 300 mg p.o. b.i.d 7 days" and the supply has 150 mg tablets of trandate, how many tablets are dispensed?
40. How many grams of dimenhydrinate are required to compound the following?

    ℞

    Dimenhydrinate
    Pantothenic acid aa 30 mg
    Thiamine HCl 10 mg
    Calcium carbonate 100 mg
    M. Ft. cap DTD #12
    Sig. i cap qid for nausea

ANSWERS

1. Take two inhalations 4 times a day, as directed.
2. Administer two drops in each eye twice a day, as directed.
3. One tablet to be taken by mouth every day, and as needed for migraine.
4. One-half (½) tablet to be taken immediately, then one tablet 3 times a day, as directed.
5. One tablet to be taken by mouth immediately, then take 2 tablets daily.
6. Apply one patch to the upper arm or chest, once weekly, as directed.
7. One tablet to be taken by mouth twice a day after meal for 10 days.
8. One capsule to be taken by mouth twice a day for 10 days.
9. One tablet to be taken every day for 10 days.
10. Take 2 tablets immediately, then 1 tablet every day.
11. Take 1 teaspoonful by mouth 3 times a day, and 2 teaspoons at bedtime.
12. Take 1 capsule by mouth every 8 hours after meal for 7 days.
13. Two capsules to be taken orally every 4 hours as needed for pain.
14. Apply one patch daily for 8 weeks.
15. Mix a teaspoonful in glassful of orange juice and drink.
16. Take 1 teaspoonful 3 times a day and when needed for diarrhea.
17. Take 2 inhalations every 4 to 6 hours as directed.
18. One tablet to be taken by mouth twice a day between meals.
19. One teaspoonful to be taken by mouth every 6 hours for 10 days.
20. Two tablets to be taken orally 3 times a day as directed.
21. Take 1 tablet twice a day before meals and 1 tablet at bedtime.
22. Take 1 tablet twice a day until all finished.
23. Insert 1 applicatorful into vagina daily at bedtime for 7 days.
24. Apply ½ inch into affected eye(s) 2-3 times a day, as directed.
25. Take 1 tablet 4 times a day for 5 days as directed.
26. Inject 10 units subcutaneously twice a day. The medication will last 100 days.
27. 0.7 mL
28. 6.5 g
29. Two drops in each ear three times a day and when necessary.
30. 26 g. One tablet to be taken every 8 hours and when necessary for pain.
31. 9750 mg. Take 1 every 6 hours as necessary for pain.
32. 1 mL
33. 18 tablets. Two tablets to be taken by mouth 3 times daily.
34. 80 tablets. Two tablets (500 mg) to be taken 4 times a day before meal.
35. 65 mg tablets
36. 8 days
37. 20 tablets
38. 4 mL
39. 28 tablets
40. 0.36 g of dimenhydrinate. Mix to make capsules. 12 such doses to be given.

6 Identifying Prescription Errors and Omissions

In the course of pharmacy practice, unintentional mistakes in the interpretation of prescriptions and dispensing of medications do happen. However, they should be minimized because of the risk to patients and huge liabilities in some cases. Most common mistakes include the following:

- The patient either receives the medication incorrectly or fails to receive it altogether.
- Prescriptions can include such erroneous information as the wrong patient, incorrect medication, inappropriate dose, wrong time, wrong route of administration, and wrong rate of administration. For example, the profile of a patient shows that he is allergic to sulfa drugs, and yet he receives Bactrim®, a sulfa drug, by error.

To prevent prescription or medication errors, it is a good practice to follow the "five rights principle" as a check:

- The right medication
- The right dose
- To right patient
- At the right time
- By the right (correct) route of administration.

The following guideline may be helpful to a pharmacist for filling prescriptions:

- Make sure that all the information required to fill the prescription is present. A systematic, step-by-step checking would be very helpful.
- Make sure that the information is correctly transferred to the prescription label.
- Make sure that the correct drug is being dispensed, whether generic or brand.
- Make sure that the DEA number is verified. This verification is especially important when controlled drugs are involved. The procedure for verification is as follows:

VERIFICATION OF THE DEA NUMBER

DEA numbers are nine-digit, specially-assigned numbers that can easily be verified in most cases. The first two of the nine digits are letters that are usually derived from the registrant's last name, business name, street address, etc. However, the third to the ninth positions from left represent a seven-digit number that can be verified. To understand the procedure, an example of DEA # AB 1359620 verification is provided below:

1. Add the first, third, and fifth digits of the seven-digit number following the letters, i.e., $1 + 5 + 6 = 12$.
2. Add the second, fourth, and sixth numbers and multiply the resultant sum by two, i.e., $3 + 9 + 2 = 14$ and $14 \times 2 = 28$.
3. Add the results of step 1 and step 2, i.e., $12 + 28 = 40$.
4. The rightmost digit is zero here. The seventh or the last digit of the DEA number is also zero.

If a DEA number follows the above rule of matching the right digit, it is most likely a genuine number. If a number doesn't match the above number, it could be an illegal prescription and the pharmacist or the nurse should verify it further by contacting the appropriate authorities. The first two letters are not easily verifiable.

A few examples of prescription errors are provided in Figure 6.1 to Figure 6.3.

EXAMPLE 1

Chris Ferell, M.D.
911 Hollywood Avenue
Detroit, MI-71208
Phone No. 555-1234

Name : John Doe **Age**: 70
Address: 96 Havana Blvd., MI-71208 **Date**: 2/28/03

℞

Flagyl 500 mg

Sig: i tab tid, 7 days

REFILL None

DAW

C. Ferell
DEA # AD 7973142

NORTHEAST PHARMACY
169 Hillside Avenue
Monroe, LA 71206 555-0342

℞ # 123456 Date: 2/28/03
Doe, John
911 Hollywood Ave
Take one tablet three times a day for seven days
Metronidazole 500 mg #40
Refill 1 C. Ferell, M.D.

FIGURE 6.1 Prescription and label for Example 1.

Errors in Example 1

1. Patient's address is wrong.
2. Number of tablets $= 3 \times 7 = 21$ and not 40.
3. Prescription shows no refill, and the label shows one refill.
4. The DEA number is wrong.

EXAMPLE 2

Pat Reno
96 Alonzo Drive
Miami, FL-71208
Phone No. 555-1234

Name : Baby Starks **Age**: 6 mo.
Address: 96 Havana Blvd., FL-71208 **Date**: 2/29/02

℞
Vantin 100 mg

Sig: 3-ss bid, 7 days

REFILL None

DAW

PReno

NORTHEAST PHARMACY
169 Hillside Avenue
Monroe, LA 71206 555-0342

℞ # 123456 Date: 2/29/01
Starks, Baby
96 Havana Blvd.
Take one-half tablet twice daily for seven days
Vantin 100 mg tablets
Refill 1 P. Reno

FIGURE 6.2 Prescription and label for Example 2.

Errors in Example 2

1. No qualifications for Pat Reno. He is not authorized to prescribe the medication.
2. Wrong date on the label.
3. The doctor meant Vantin suspension (100 mg/5 mL), which is clear from the *signa*. Tablets are a wrong choice for an infant.
4. *Signa* should be one-half teaspoonful twice daily for seven days.
5. No refills. The label shows one.
6. Registration number or DEA is missing for Pat Reno.

EXAMPLE 3

Doc Rogers, M.D.
12 Progress Drive
Amarillo, TX-79106
Phone No. 555-1234

Name : Jackie Bushnell **Age**: 58 yrs
Address: 20 Main Street, Amarillo **Date**: 7/9/01

℞
Fiorinal with Codeine
 # 40

Sig: ii caps, q4h daily

REFILL 1

DAW _

DRogers
DEA # DR1234567

FIGURE 6.3 Prescription for Example 3.

Errors in Example 3

1. Jackie Bushnell is allergic to aspirin. Therefore, Fiorinal® with codeine, which contains aspirin, should not be given.
2. Jackie Bushnell is taking Tylenol® #3, which contains codeine, since 7/7/01. Probably the codeine preparation is being abused, and Dr. Rogers should be informed.

PRACTICE PRESCRIPTIONS FOR ERRORS AND OMISSIONS

1.

Howard Huxtable, M.D.
20 Sheldon Street
Amarillo, TX-79119
Phone No. 555-1234

Name : John Doe **Age**: 30
Address: 96 Progress Drive, TX-79119 **Date**: 2/28/02

℞

Zantac 300 mg

Sig: i bid, 15 days

REFILL None

DAW √

HHuxtable
DEA # AD 7973142

NORTHEAST PHARMACY
822 Coulter Street
Amarillo, TX-79106 555-0342

℞ # 123456 Date: 2/28/02
Doe, John
96 Progress Dr.
Take one tablet at bed time
Ranitidine 300 mg # 40
H. Huxtable, M.D.

2.

Howard Huxtable, M.D.
20 Sheldon Street
Amarillo, TX-79119
Phone No. 555-1234

Name : Alice Smith **Age**: 8 mo.
Address: 96 Progress Drive, TX-79119 **Date**: 1/18/02

℞

Amoxil 250 mg/tablet

Disp. # 28

Sig: i tab q6h until finished

REFILL

DAW

HHuxtable
DEA # AD 7973142

NORTHEAST PHARMACY
822 Coulter Street
Amarillo, TX-79106 555-0342

℞ # 123456 Date: 1/18/02
Smith, Alice
96 Progress Dr.
Take one tablet every six hours until Friday
Amoxicillin 250 mg
H. Huxtable, M.D.

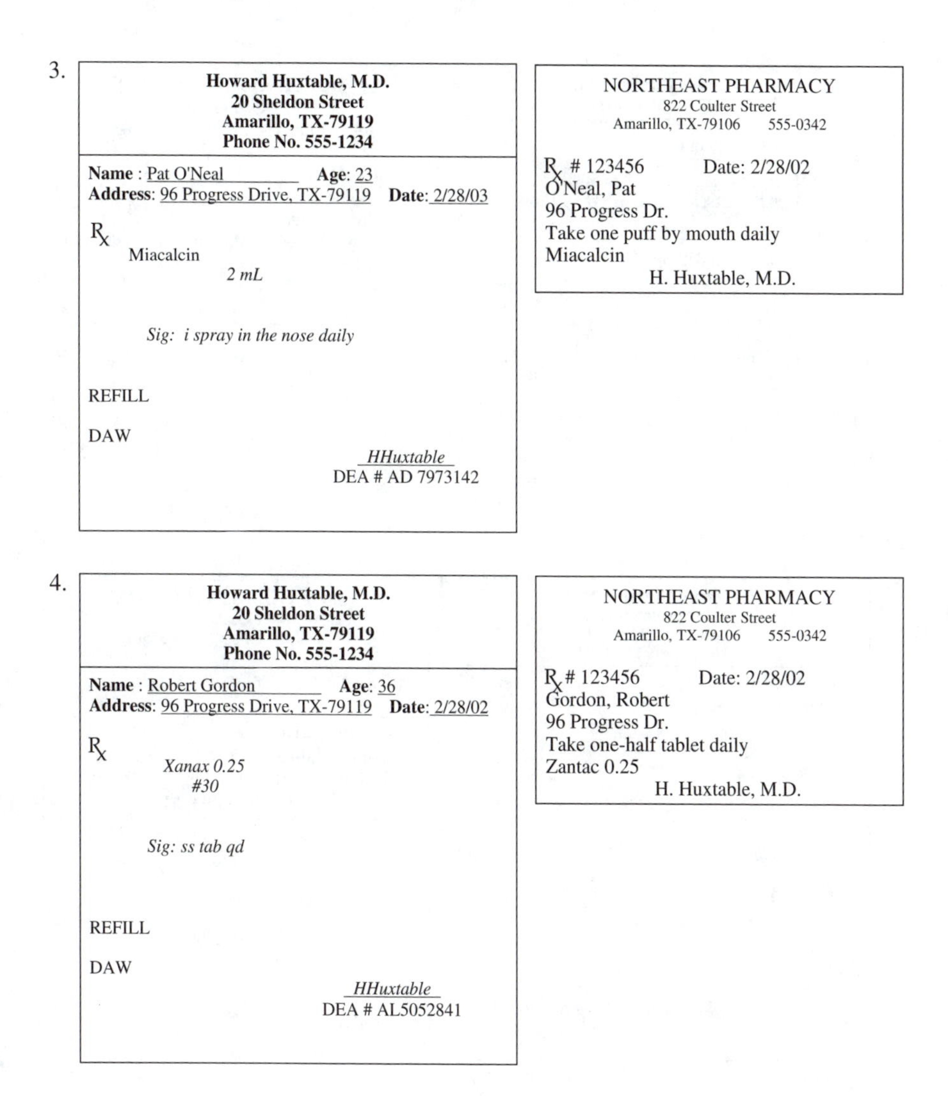

3.

Howard Huxtable, M.D.
20 Sheldon Street
Amarillo, TX-79119
Phone No. 555-1234

Name : Pat O'Neal **Age**: 23
Address: 96 Progress Drive, TX-79119 **Date**: 2/28/03

℞
Miacalcin
2 mL

Sig: i spray in the nose daily

REFILL

DAW

HHuxtable
DEA # AD 7973142

NORTHEAST PHARMACY
822 Coulter Street
Amarillo, TX-79106 555-0342

℞ # 123456 Date: 2/28/02
O'Neal, Pat
96 Progress Dr.
Take one puff by mouth daily
Miacalcin
H. Huxtable, M.D.

4.

Howard Huxtable, M.D.
20 Sheldon Street
Amarillo, TX-79119
Phone No. 555-1234

Name : Robert Gordon **Age**: 36
Address: 96 Progress Drive, TX-79119 **Date**: 2/28/02

℞
Xanax 0.25
#30

Sig: ss tab qd

REFILL

DAW

HHuxtable
DEA # AL5052841

NORTHEAST PHARMACY
822 Coulter Street
Amarillo, TX-79106 555-0342

℞ # 123456 Date: 2/28/02
Gordon, Robert
96 Progress Dr.
Take one-half tablet daily
Zantac 0.25
H. Huxtable, M.D.

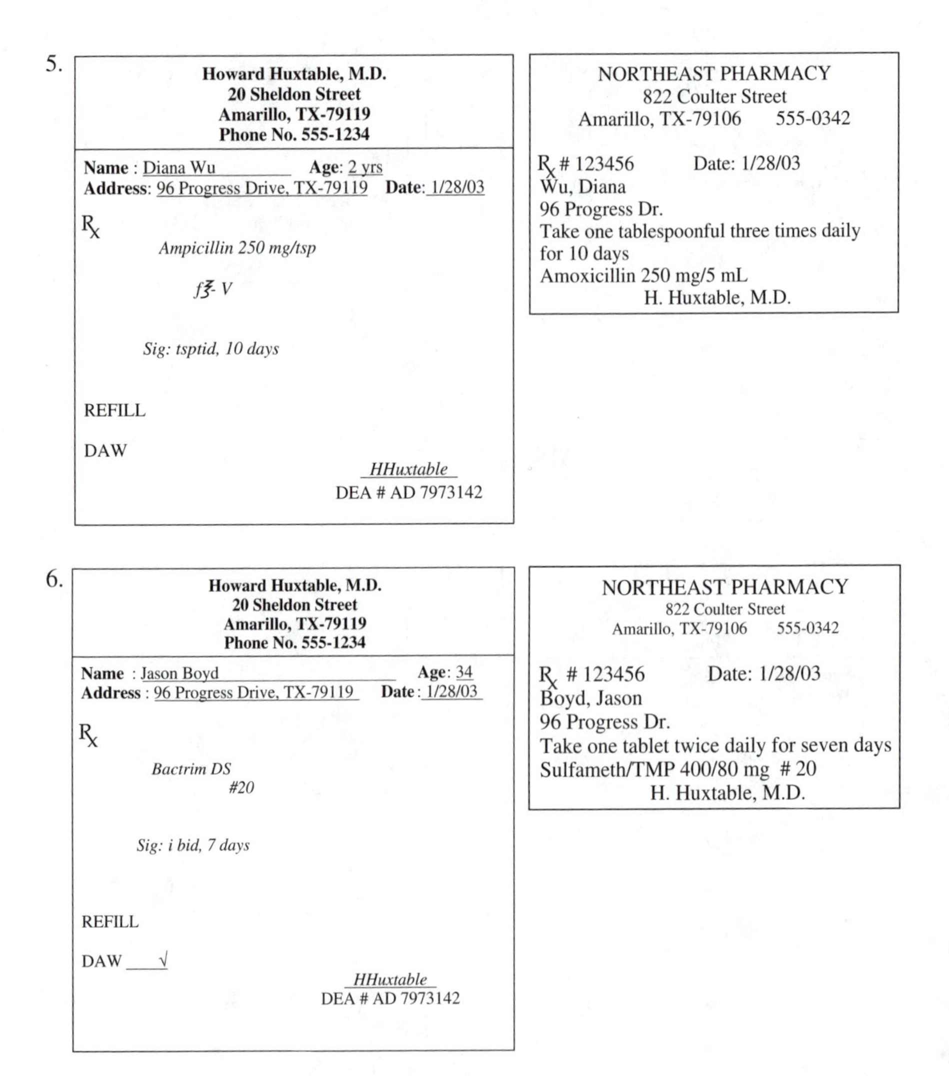

5.

Howard Huxtable, M.D.
20 Sheldon Street
Amarillo, TX-79119
Phone No. 555-1234

Name : Diana Wu **Age**: 2 yrs
Address: 96 Progress Drive, TX-79119 **Date**: 1/28/03

℞

Ampicillin 250 mg/tsp

f℥- V

Sig: tsptid, 10 days

REFILL

DAW

HHuxtable
DEA # AD 7973142

NORTHEAST PHARMACY
822 Coulter Street
Amarillo, TX-79106 555-0342

℞ # 123456 Date: 1/28/03
Wu, Diana
96 Progress Dr.
Take one tablespoonful three times daily for 10 days
Amoxicillin 250 mg/5 mL
H. Huxtable, M.D.

6.

Howard Huxtable, M.D.
20 Sheldon Street
Amarillo, TX-79119
Phone No. 555-1234

Name : Jason Boyd **Age**: 34
Address : 96 Progress Drive, TX-79119 **Date** : 1/28/03

℞

Bactrim DS
#20

Sig: i bid, 7 days

REFILL

DAW √

HHuxtable
DEA # AD 7973142

NORTHEAST PHARMACY
822 Coulter Street
Amarillo, TX-79106 555-0342

℞ # 123456 Date: 1/28/03
Boyd, Jason
96 Progress Dr.
Take one tablet twice daily for seven days
Sulfameth/TMP 400/80 mg # 20
H. Huxtable, M.D.

7.

Howard Huxtable, M.D.
20 Sheldon Street
Amarillo, TX-79119
Phone No. 555-1234

Name : Alicia Bedell **Age**: 4 mo.
Address : 96 Progress Drive, TX-79119 **Date** : 1/25/03

℞

ASA Suppositories 2 gr
#10

Sig: In. rect q4h, prn fever over 101 °

REFILL

DAW

HHuxtable
DEA # AD 7973142

NORTHEAST PHARMACY
822 Coulter Street
Amarillo, TX-79106 555-0342

℞ # 123456 Date: 1/25/03
Bedell, Alicia
96 Progress Dr.
Insert one suppository rectally four times daily for fever over 101°
APAP Suppositories 2 gr #10
H. Huxtable, M.D.

8. **Medication profile and a prescription**

Evelyn Bradley
20 Main Street
Monroe, LA 71201 Allergy: Penicillin, Sulfa, Cephalosporins

Date	Dr.	_#	Patient	Drug
3/1/02	Quinn	12340	Evelyn	Baycol 0.2 mg #100, 1 daily
5/6/02	Quinn	12350	Evelyn	Amaryl 2 mg #60, 1 qd
7/7/02	Quinn	12369	Evelyn	Tylenol #3 # 30, ii tid, prn

Doc Rogers, M.D.
12 Desiard Street
Amarillo, TX-79119
Phone No. 555-1234

Name : Evelyn Bradley **Age**: 18 yrs
Address : 20 Main Street, Monroe **Date** : 7/9/02

℞

Omnicef 300 mg

Sig: ibid, 7 days

REFILL 1

DAW √

DRogers
DEA #DR1234567

NORTHEAST PHARMACY
822 Coulter Street
Amarillo, TX-79106 555-0342

℞ # 123456 Date: 7/9/02
Bradley, Evelyn
20 Main St
Take one tablet twice daily for seven days
Omniceff 300 mg # 18
D. Rogers, M.D.

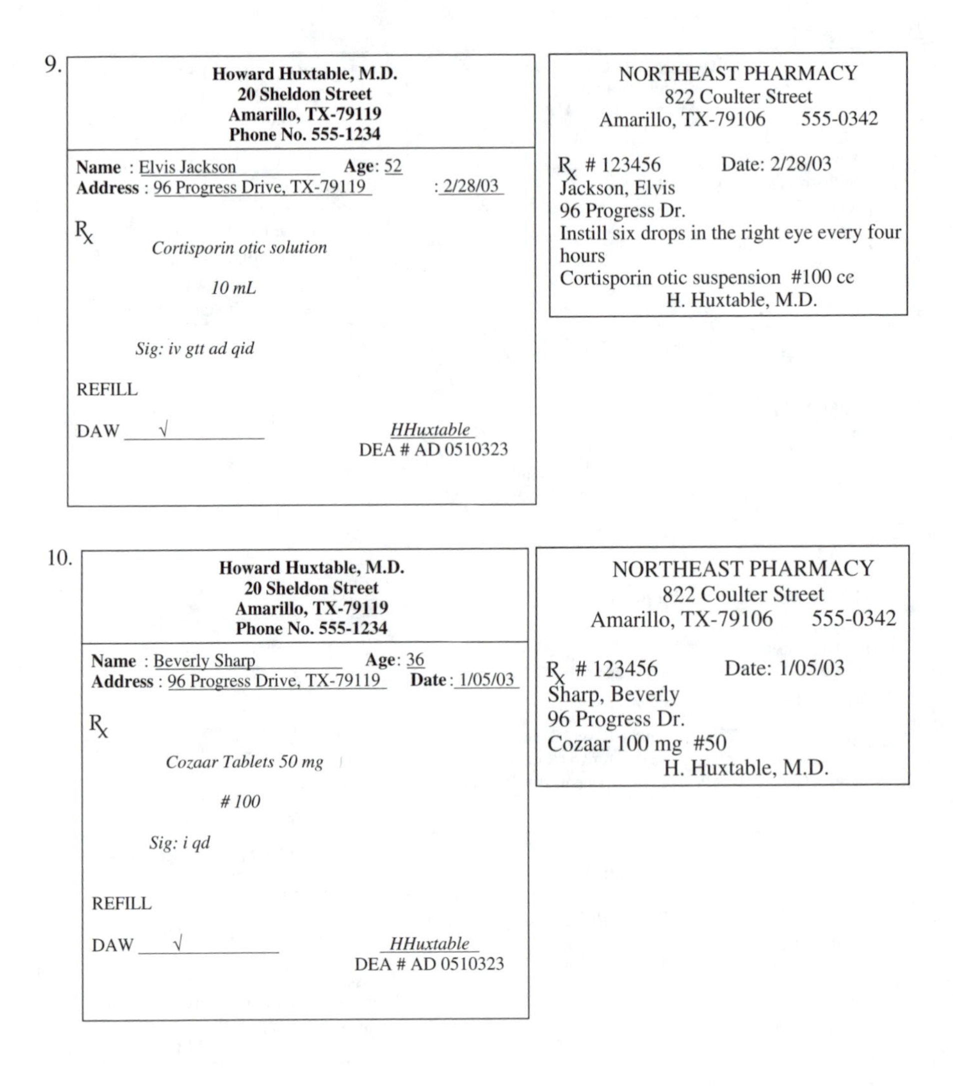

9.

Howard Huxtable, M.D.
20 Sheldon Street
Amarillo, TX-79119
Phone No. 555-1234

Name : Elvis Jackson **Age**: 52
Address : 96 Progress Drive, TX-79119 : 2/28/03

℞

Cortisporin otic solution

10 mL

Sig: iv gtt ad qid

REFILL

DAW √

HHuxtable
DEA # AD 0510323

NORTHEAST PHARMACY
822 Coulter Street
Amarillo, TX-79106 555-0342

℞ # 123456 Date: 2/28/03
Jackson, Elvis
96 Progress Dr.
Instill six drops in the right eye every four hours
Cortisporin otic suspension #100 cc
H. Huxtable, M.D.

10.

Howard Huxtable, M.D.
20 Sheldon Street
Amarillo, TX-79119
Phone No. 555-1234

Name : Beverly Sharp **Age**: 36
Address : 96 Progress Drive, TX-79119 **Date** : 1/05/03

℞

Cozaar Tablets 50 mg

 # 100

Sig: i qd

REFILL

DAW √

HHuxtable
DEA # AD 0510323

NORTHEAST PHARMACY
822 Coulter Street
Amarillo, TX-79106 555-0342

℞ # 123456 Date: 1/05/03
Sharp, Beverly
96 Progress Dr.
Cozaar 100 mg #50
H. Huxtable, M.D.

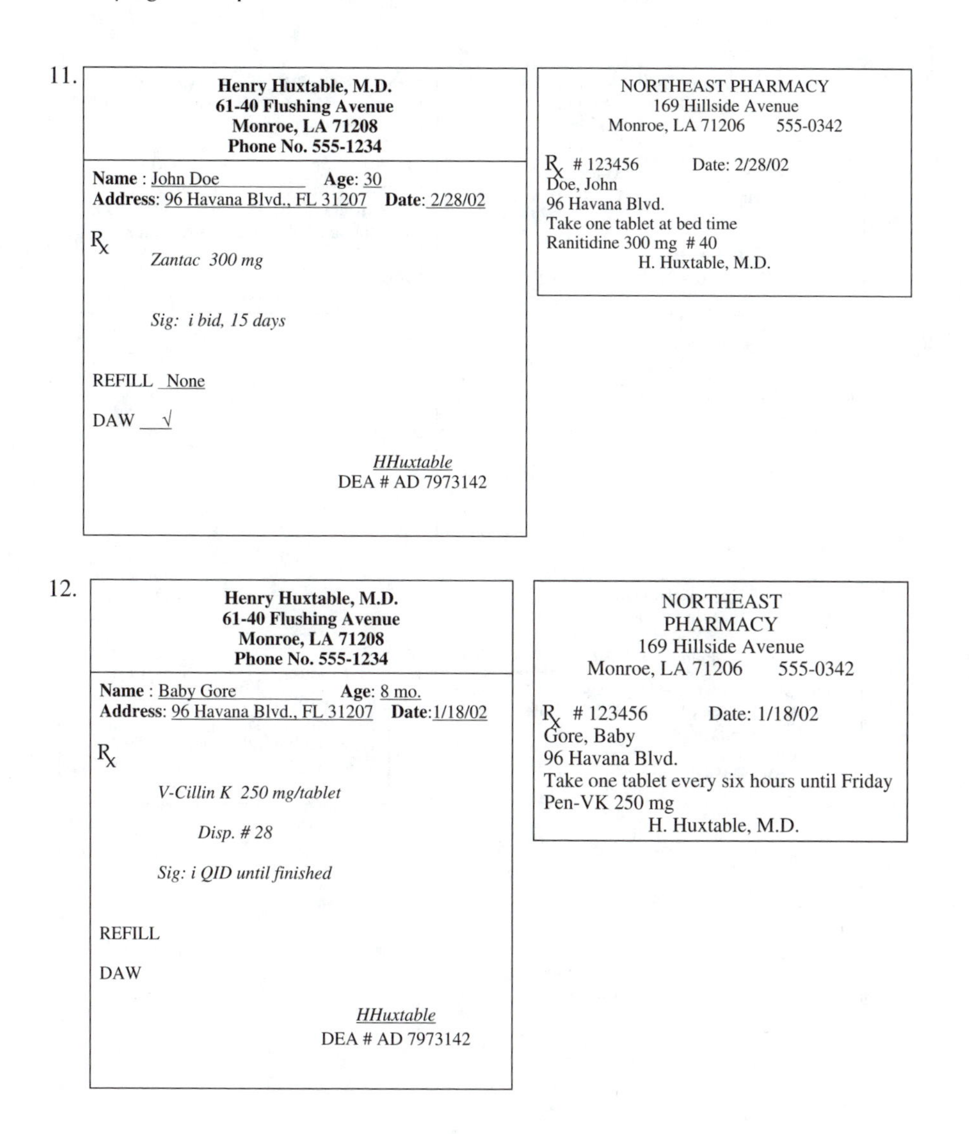

11.

Henry Huxtable, M.D.
61-40 Flushing Avenue
Monroe, LA 71208
Phone No. 555-1234

Name : John Doe **Age**: 30
Address: 96 Havana Blvd., FL 31207 **Date**: 2/28/02

℞ *Zantac 300 mg*

Sig: i bid, 15 days

REFILL None

DAW √

HHuxtable
DEA # AD 7973142

NORTHEAST PHARMACY
169 Hillside Avenue
Monroe, LA 71206 555-0342

℞ # 123456 Date: 2/28/02
Doe, John
96 Havana Blvd.
Take one tablet at bed time
Ranitidine 300 mg # 40
H. Huxtable, M.D.

12.

Henry Huxtable, M.D.
61-40 Flushing Avenue
Monroe, LA 71208
Phone No. 555-1234

Name : Baby Gore **Age**: 8 mo.
Address: 96 Havana Blvd., FL 31207 **Date**:1/18/02

℞ *V-Cillin K 250 mg/tablet*

Disp. # 28

Sig: i QID until finished

REFILL

DAW

HHuxtable
DEA # AD 7973142

NORTHEAST PHARMACY
169 Hillside Avenue
Monroe, LA 71206 555-0342

℞ # 123456 Date: 1/18/02
Gore, Baby
96 Havana Blvd.
Take one tablet every six hours until Friday
Pen-VK 250 mg
H. Huxtable, M.D.

13.

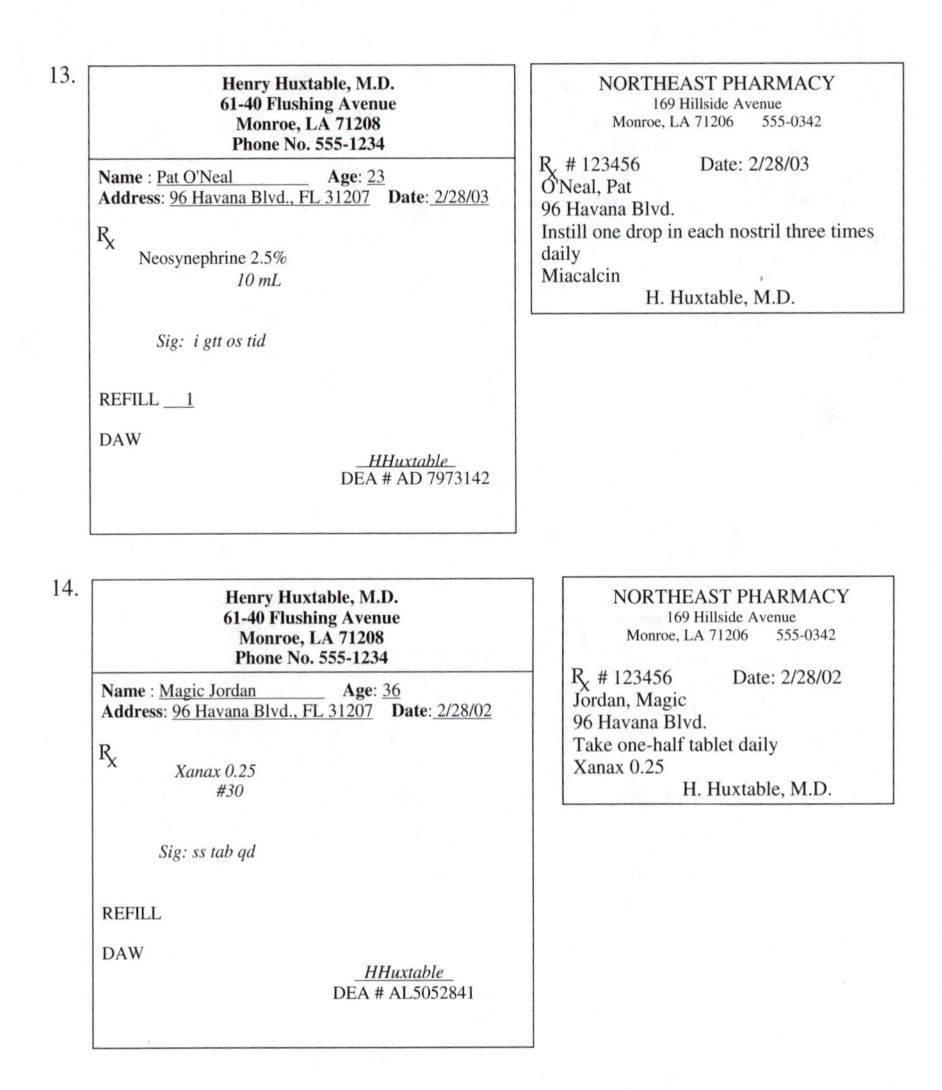

Henry Huxtable, M.D.
61-40 Flushing Avenue
Monroe, LA 71208
Phone No. 555-1234

Name : Pat O'Neal **Age**: 23
Address: 96 Havana Blvd., FL 31207 **Date**: 2/28/03

℞

Neosynephrine 2.5%
10 mL

Sig: i gtt os tid

REFILL 1

DAW

HHuxtable
DEA # AD 7973142

NORTHEAST PHARMACY
169 Hillside Avenue
Monroe, LA 71206 555-0342

℞ # 123456 Date: 2/28/03
O'Neal, Pat
96 Havana Blvd.
Instill one drop in each nostril three times daily
Miacalcin
H. Huxtable, M.D.

14.

Henry Huxtable, M.D.
61-40 Flushing Avenue
Monroe, LA 71208
Phone No. 555-1234

Name : Magic Jordan **Age**: 36
Address: 96 Havana Blvd., FL 31207 **Date**: 2/28/02

℞

Xanax 0.25
#30

Sig: ss tab qd

REFILL

DAW

HHuxtable
DEA # AL5052841

NORTHEAST PHARMACY
169 Hillside Avenue
Monroe, LA 71206 555-0342

℞ # 123456 Date: 2/28/02
Jordan, Magic
96 Havana Blvd.
Take one-half tablet daily
Xanax 0.25
H. Huxtable, M.D.

15.

Henry Huxtable, M.D.
61-40 Flushing Avenue
Monroe, LA 71208
Phone No. 555-1234

Name : Gill Bates **Age**: 2 yrs
Address: 96 Havana Blvd., FL 31207 **Date**: 1/28/03

℞

Ampicillin 250 mg/tsp

f℥ V

Sig: tsptid, 10 days

REFILL

DAW ______________ *HHuxtable*
DEA# AD 7973142

NORTHEAST PHARMACY
169 Hillside Avenue
Monroe, LA 71206 555-0342

℞ # 123456 Date: 1/28/03
Khan, Adnan
96 Havana Blvd.
Take one tablespoonful three times daily for 10 days
Amoxicillin 250 mg/5 mL
H. Huxtable, M.D.

16.

Henry Huxtable, M.D.
61-40 Flushing Avenue
Monroe, LA 71208
Phone No. 555-1234

Name : Robin Williams **Age**: 34
Address : 96 Havana Blvd., FL 31207 **Date** : 1/28/03

℞

Septra DS
#20

Sig: i bid, 7 days

REFILL 1

DAW √

HHuxtable
DEA # AD 7973142

NORTHEAST PHARMACY
169 Hillside Avenue
Monroe, LA 71206 555-0342

℞ # 123456 Date: 1/28/03
Williams, Robin
96 Havana Blvd.
Take one tablet twice daily for seven days
Sulfameth/TMP 400/80 mg # 20
H. Huxtable, M.D.

17.

Henry Huxtable, M.D.
61-40 Flushing Avenue
Monroe, LA 71208
Phone No. 555-1234

Name : Mary Green **Age**: 4 mo.
Address : 96 Havana Blvd., FL 31207 **Date**: 1/25/03

℞

APAP Suppositories 1 gr
#10

Sig: In. rect q4h, prn fever over 101°

REFILL

DAW

HHuxtable
DEA # AD7973142

NORTHEAST PHARMACY
169 Hillside Avenue
Monroe, LA 71206 555-0342

℞ # 123456 Date: 1/25/03
Green, Mary
96 Havana Blvd.
Insert one suppository rectally four times daily for fever over 101°
ASA Suppositories 2 gr #10
H. Huxtable, M.D.

18. **Medication profile and a prescription**

Evelyn Monroe
20 Main Street
Monroe, LA 71201 Allergy: Penicillin, Sulfa

Date	Dr.	_ #	Patient	Drug
3/1/02	Quinn	12340	Evelyn	Synthroid 0.2 mg #100, 1 daily
5/6/02	Quinn	12350	Evelyn	Hygroton 2.5 mg #70, 1 qd
7/8/02	Quinn	12369	Evelyn	Tylenol #3 # 30, ii tid, prn

Doc Rogers, M.D.
12 Desiard Street
Monroe, LA-71208
Phone No. 555-1234

Name : Evelyn Monroe **Age**: 18 yrs
Address : 20 Main Street, Monroe **Date**: 7/9/02

Fiorinal with Codeine # 40

Sig: iqid, 7 days

REFILL 1

DAW √

DRogers
DEA # DR1234567

NORTHEAST PHARMACY
169 Hillside Avenue
Monroe, LA 71206 555-0342

123456 Date: 7/9/02
Monroe, Evelyn
20 Main St
Take one tablet four times daily for seven days
Fiorinal with Codeine # 28
D. Rogers, M.D.

19.

Henry Huxtable, M.D.
61-40 Flushing Avenue
Monroe, LA 71208
Phone No. 555-1234

Name : Elvis Jackson **Age**: 52
Address : 96 Havana Blvd., FL 31207 **Date** : 2/28/03

℞

Cortisporin otic solution

10 mL

Sig: VI gtt ad qid

REFILL

DAW √

HHuxtable
DEA # AD 0510323

NORTHEAST PHARMACY
169 Hillside Avenue
Monroe, LA 71206 555-0342

℞ # 123456 Date: 2/28/03
Jackson, Elvis
96 Havana Blvd.
Instill six drops in the right eye every four hours
Cortisporin otic suspension #100 cc
H. Huxtable, M.D.

20.

Henry Huxtable, M.D.
61-40 Flushing Avenue
Monroe, LA 71208
Phone No. 555-1234

Name : Beverly Sharp **Age**: 36
Address : 96 Havana Blvd., FL 31207 **Date** : 1/05/03

℞

Tenormin Tablets 50 mg

 # 100

Sig: i qd

REFILL 5X

DAW √

HHuxtable
DEA # AD 0510323

NORTHEAST PHARMACY
169 Hillside Avenue
Monroe, LA 71206 555-0342

℞# 123456 Date: 1/05/03
Sharp, Beverly
96 Havana Blvd.
Tenormin 100 mg #50
H. Huxtable, M.D.

21.

Henry Huxtable, M.D.
61-40 Flushing Avenue
Monroe, LA 71208
Phone No. 555-1234

Name : John Doe **Age**: 30
Address: 96 Havana Blvd., FL 31207 **Date**: 2/28/02

℞

Zantac 300 mg

Sig: i bid, 15 days

REFILL None

DAW √

HHuxtable
DEA # AD 7973142

NORTHEAST PHARMACY
169 Hillside Avenue
Monroe, LA 71206 555-0342

℞ # 123456 Date: 2/28/02
Doe, John
96 Havana Blvd.
Take one tablet twice daily for fifteen days
Ranitidine 150 mg # 80
H. Huxtable, M.D.

22.

Henry Huxtable, M.D.
61-40 Flushing Avenue
Monroe, LA 71208
Phone No. 555-1234

Name : Baby Gore **Age**: 8 mo.
Address: 96 Havana Blvd., FL 31207 **Date**:1/18/02

℞

V-Cillin K 250 mg/tablet

Disp. # 28

Sig: i QID until finished

REFILL

DAW

HHuxtable
DEA # AD 7973142

NORTHEAST PHARMACY
169 Hillside Avenue
Monroe, LA 71206 555-0342

℞ # 123456 Date: 1/18/02
Gore, Baby
61-40 flushing Ave
Take one tablet every six hours until Friday
Pen-VK 250 mg
H. Huxtable, M.D.

23.

Henry Huxtable, M.D.
61-40 Flushing Avenue
Monroe, LA 71208
Phone No. 555-1234

Name : Pat O'Neal **Age**: 23
Address: 96 Havana Blvd., FL 31207 **Date**: 2/28/03

Rx
Neosynephrine 2.5%
10 mL

Sig: i gtt os tid

REFILL 1

DAW

HHuxtable
DEA # AD 7973142

NORTHEAST PHARMACY
169 Hillside Avenue
Monroe, LA 71206 555-0342

Rx # 123456 Date: 2/28/03
O'Neal, Pat
96 Havana Blvd.
Instill one drop in each nostril three times daily
Neosporine 1.5%
H. Huxtable, M.D.

24.

Henry Huxtable, M.D.
61-40 Flushing Avenue
Monroe, LA 71208
Phone No. 555-1234

Name : Magic Jordan **Age**: 36
Address: 96 Havana Blvd., FL 31207 **Date**: 2/28/02

Rx
Xanax 0.25
#30

Sig: ss tab qd

REFILL

DAW

HHuxtable
DEA #AL5052841

NORTHEAST PHARMACY
169 Hillside Avenue
Monroe, LA 71206 555-0342

Rx # 123456 Date: 2/28/02
Jordan, Magic
96 Havana Blvd.
Take one-half tablet daily
Xanax 0.5
H. Huxtable, M.D.

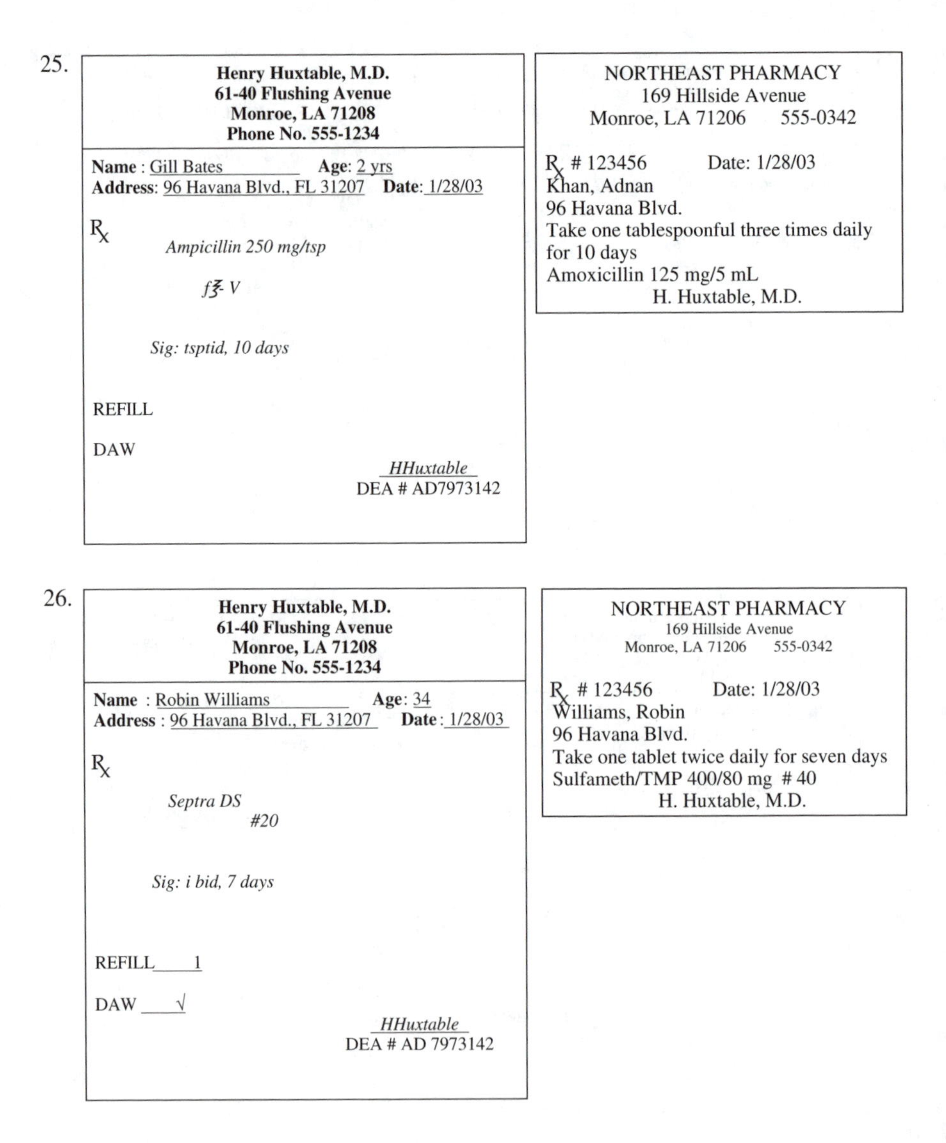

25.

Henry Huxtable, M.D.
61-40 Flushing Avenue
Monroe, LA 71208
Phone No. 555-1234

Name: Gill Bates **Age**: 2 yrs
Address: 96 Havana Blvd., FL 31207 **Date**: 1/28/03

℞

Ampicillin 250 mg/tsp

f℥ V

Sig: tsptid, 10 days

REFILL

DAW

HHuxtable
DEA # AD7973142

NORTHEAST PHARMACY
169 Hillside Avenue
Monroe, LA 71206 555-0342

℞ # 123456 Date: 1/28/03
Khan, Adnan
96 Havana Blvd.
Take one tablespoonful three times daily for 10 days
Amoxicillin 125 mg/5 mL
H. Huxtable, M.D.

26.

Henry Huxtable, M.D.
61-40 Flushing Avenue
Monroe, LA 71208
Phone No. 555-1234

Name: Robin Williams **Age**: 34
Address: 96 Havana Blvd., FL 31207 **Date**: 1/28/03

℞

Septra DS
#20

Sig: i bid, 7 days

REFILL 1

DAW √

HHuxtable
DEA # AD 7973142

NORTHEAST PHARMACY
169 Hillside Avenue
Monroe, LA 71206 555-0342

℞ # 123456 Date: 1/28/03
Williams, Robin
96 Havana Blvd.
Take one tablet twice daily for seven days
Sulfameth/TMP 400/80 mg # 40
H. Huxtable, M.D.

27.

Henry Huxtable 61-40 Flushing Avenue Monroe, LA 71208 Phone No. 555-1234
Name : Mary Green **Age**: 4 mo. **Address** : 96 Havana Blvd., FL 31207 **Date**: 1/25/03 ℞ *APAP Suppositories 1 gr* *#10* *Sig: In. rect q4h, prn fever over 101°* REFILL DAW *HHuxtable*

NORTHEAST PHARMACY
169 Hillside Avenue
Monroe, LA 71206 555-0342

℞ # 123456 Date: 1/25/03
Green, Mary
96 Havana Blvd.
Insert one suppository rectally four times daily for fever over 101°
ASA Suppositories 2 gr #10
H. Huxtable

28. **Medication profile and a prescription**

Evelyn Monroe
20 Main Street
Monroe, LA 71201 Allergy: Sulfa, Codeine

Date	Dr.	_#	Patient	Drug
3/1/02	Quinn	12340	Evelyn	Synthroid 0.2 mg #100, 1 daily
5/6/02	Quinn	12350	Evelyn	Hygroton 2.5 mg #70, 1 qd

Doc Rogers, M.D. 12 Desiard Street Monroe, LA-71208 Phone No. 555-1234
Name : Evelyn Monroe **Age**: 18 yrs **Address** : 20 Main Street, Monroe : 7/9/02 ℞ *Fiorinal with Codeine # 40* *Sig: iqid, 7 days* REFILL 1 DAW √ *DRogers* DEA # DR1234567

NORTHEAST PHARMACY
169 Hillside Avenue
Monroe, LA 71206 555-0342

℞ # 123456 Date: 7/9/02
Monroe, Evelyn
20 Main St
Take one tablet four times daily for seven days
Fiorinal with Codeine # 28
D. Rogers, M.D.

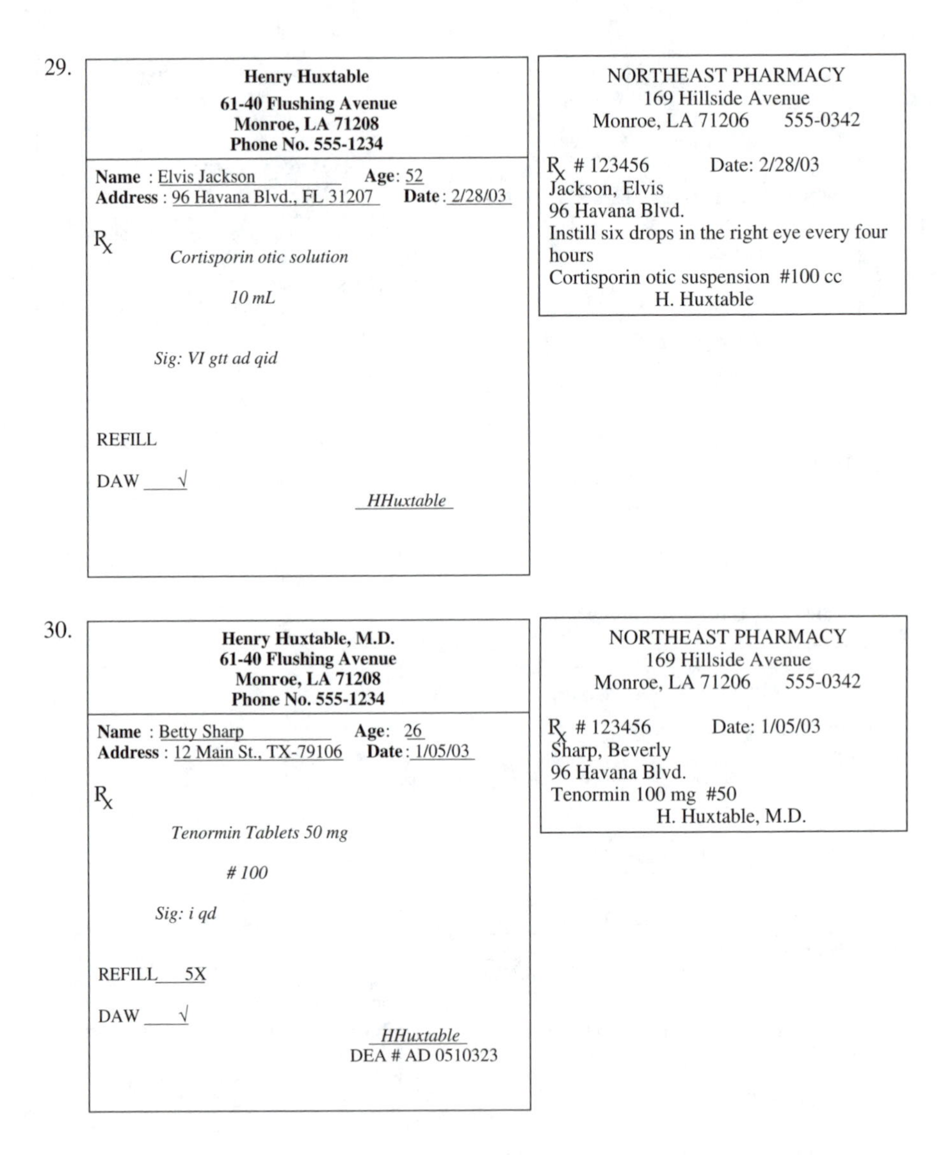

29.

Henry Huxtable
61-40 Flushing Avenue
Monroe, LA 71208
Phone No. 555-1234

Name : Elvis Jackson **Age**: 52
Address : 96 Havana Blvd., FL 31207 **Date**: 2/28/03

℞

Cortisporin otic solution

10 mL

Sig: VI gtt ad qid

REFILL

DAW √

HHuxtable

NORTHEAST PHARMACY
169 Hillside Avenue
Monroe, LA 71206 555-0342

℞ # 123456 Date: 2/28/03
Jackson, Elvis
96 Havana Blvd.
Instill six drops in the right eye every four hours
Cortisporin otic suspension #100 cc
H. Huxtable

30.

Henry Huxtable, M.D.
61-40 Flushing Avenue
Monroe, LA 71208
Phone No. 555-1234

Name : Betty Sharp **Age**: 26
Address : 12 Main St., TX-79106 **Date**: 1/05/03

℞

Tenormin Tablets 50 mg

 # 100

Sig: i qd

REFILL 5X

DAW √

HHuxtable
DEA # AD 0510323

NORTHEAST PHARMACY
169 Hillside Avenue
Monroe, LA 71206 555-0342

℞ # 123456 Date: 1/05/03
Sharp, Beverly
96 Havana Blvd.
Tenormin 100 mg #50
H. Huxtable, M.D.

ANSWERS

1. a. Generic is dispensed instead of brand
   b. 30 tablets should be given and not 40
   c. Wrong DEA number
   d. Wrong instructions
2. a. Wrong dosage form for an eight-month-old baby
   b. Wrong instructions: Until finished and not until Friday
   c. Wrong DEA number
3. a. Wrong instructions on the label
   b. Wrong date on the label
   c. Wrong DEA number
4. a. Wrong drug
   b. Wrong strength because Zantac® is unavailable in that strength
   c. Wrong DEA number
5. a. Wrong medication
   b. Wrong directions
   c. Wrong DEA number
6. a. Wrong medication strength
   b. Generic not allowed
   c. Wrong quantity of medication since the strength is reduced to one-half
   d. Wrong DEA number
7. a. Wrong medication (APAP and not ASA)
   b. Wrong directions: Every four hours and not four times
   c. Wrong DEA number
8. a. Pateint is allergic to cyclosporines. Omniceff should be avoided.
   b. Wrong quantity of medication. 14 should be given and not 18.
   c. Wrong DEA number
   d. One refill
9. a. Otic solution and not suspension
   b. Wrong directions; 4 drops and not 6 drops, right ear and not right eye
   c. Four times and not every four hours
   d. Wrong quantity: 10 cc and not 100 cc
   e. Wrong DEA number
10. a. Wrong strength: 50 mg and not 100 mg
    b. Wrong quantity: 100 and not 50
    c. Directions are missing
    d. Wrong DEA number
11. a. Generic is dispensed instead of brand
    b. 30 tablets of 300 mg should be given and not 40
    c. Wrong DEA number
    d. Wrong instructions
12. a. Wrong dosage form for an 8-month-old baby
    b. Wrong instructions: Four times a day until finished
    c. Wrong DEA number

13. a. Wrong instructions on the label
    b. Wrong medication
    c. Refill missing in the prescription label
    d. Wrong DEA number
14. a. Wrong DEA number
15. a. Wrong patient
    b. Wrong medication
    c. Wrong directions
    d. Wrong DEA number
16. a. Wrong medication strength
    b. Generic not allowed
    c. Wrong quantity of medication (should be 40 for ½ strength tablets)
    d. Wrong instructions: Take two tablets twice daily for ½ strength tablets
    e. Refill missing in the label
    f. Wrong DEA number
17. a. Wrong medication (APAP and not ASA)
    b. Wrong strength
    c. Wrong directions: Every four hours and not four times
18. a. Patient is allergic to codeine: Wrong choice of the drug
    b. Number of tablets should be 28 and not 40
    c. Wrong DEA number
    d. One refill
19. a. Otic solution and not suspension
    b. Wrong directions; right ear and not right eye
    c. Four times and not every four hours
    d. Wrong quantity: 10 cc and not 100 cc
    e. Wrong DEA number
20. a. Wrong strength: 50 mg and not 100 mg
    b. Wrong quantity: 100 and not 50
    c. Directions are missing
    d. Five refills are missing
    e. Wrong DEA number
21. a. Generic is dispensed instead of brand
    b. 60 tablets of 150 mg should be given and not 80
    c. Wrong DEA number
    d. Wrong instructions for ½ strength tablets
22. a. Wrong dosage form for an 8-month-old baby
    b. Wrong address of the patient
    c. Wrong DEA number
23. a. Wrong drug
    b. Wrong instructions on the label
    c. Wrong medication strength
    d. Wrong DEA number
24. a. Wrong strength
    b. Wrong DEA number

25. a. Wrong patient
    b. Wrong medication
    c. Wrong strength
    d. Wrong directions
    e. Wrong DEA number
26. a. Wrong medication strength
    b. Generic not allowed
    c. Wrong signa instructions on the label for ½ strength tablets
    d. Wrong DEA number
27. a. Wrong medication (APAP and not ASA)
    b. Wrong strength
    c. Wrong directions: Every four hours and not four times
    d. No prescribing authority
    e. No License or DEA number
28. a. Patient is allergic to codeine; wrong drug
    b. Number of tablets should be 28 and not 40
    c. Wrong DEA number
    d. One refill
29. a. No prescribing authority
    b. Otic solution and not suspension
    c. Wrong directions; right ear and not right eye
    d. Four times and not every four hours
    e. Wrong quantity: 10 cc and not 100 cc
    f. DEA or License number is missing
30. a. Wrong patient
    b. Wrong address
    c. Wrong strength: 50 mg and not 100 mg
    d. Wrong quantity: 100 and not 50
    e. Directions are missing
    f. Five refills are missing
    g. Wrong DEA number

7 Working with Liquid Dosage Forms

A pharmacist prepares and dispenses oral liquid dosage forms routinely. The oral liquid dosage forms are mainly syrups, elixirs, and suspensions. Among these three, syrups and elixirs are homogenous (uniform concentration throughout the liquid), and suspensions are heterogeneous, where the concentration is not uniform throughout the liquid. When medicated, all these preparations contain a specific amount of drug in a given amount of liquid. The solution strength, stated on the label, may indicate the amount (in μg, mg, or g) of drug per one milliliter or multiple milliliters of solution, such as 10 mg per mL, 1.2 g per 20 mL, etc. The strength may also be expressed as g or mg per teaspoonful (or 5 mL). The strength of certain biological products may be expressed as units of activity per milliliter or milliequivalents per liter.

Syrups are concentrated aqueous solutions of sucrose or other sugar or sugar-substitute with or without added medicinal substances and flavoring agents. The formulation of a syrup contains the drug(s), a sugar, antimicrobial preservatives, colorants, and flavorants. The sugar content may vary from 60 to 85%. *Syrup, USP* (also referred to as "simple syrup") contains 85 grams of sucrose per 100 mL of syrup. Elixirs are clear oral solutions in which the vehicle is a hydroalcoholic mixture containing potent or nauseating drugs. The presence of a hydroalcoholic vehicle in an elixir makes it possible to include both water-soluble and alcohol-soluble substances in solution. Suspensions are two-phase systems consisting of finely divided particles of drug(s) dispersed in a vehicle in which the drug is insoluble or poorly soluble. Most of the suspensions of pharmaceutical interest are aqueous dispersions, available either in ready-to-use form or as dry powders to circumvent the instability of aqueous dispersions of certain drugs, such as antibiotics. At the time of dispensing, the latter types of preparations are reconstituted with water to complete the suspension. These preparations are designated in the USP as "*...for oral suspension.*"

LIQUID CALCULATIONS INVOLVING PROPORTIONS

The calculations involving proportions are highlighted in Chapter 3. For the oral liquids, the proportions method can be used to prepare a bulk formula when the strength per unit dose is given. These calculations are also called "enlargement" calculations. Opposite to enlargement calculations are the "reduction" calculations, where the formula for a bulk preparation is given and the strength per unit dose (for e.g., per teaspoonful) is calculated. Some examples of liquid calculations where proportions are used follow.

Example 1:

An elixir of phenobarbital contains 10 mg of phenobarbital in each 5 mL. How many mg would be used in preparing one liter of the elixir?

$$10 \text{ mg}/5 \text{ mL} = \text{X mg}/1000 \text{ mL}$$

$$\text{X} = 2000 \text{ mg or } 2 \text{ g, answer}$$

Example 2:

Amobarbital elixir contains 8 g of amobarbital/liter. How many milligrams of amobarbital are contained in a teaspoonful dose of the elixir?

$$8 \text{ g} = 8000 \text{ mg}$$

$$8000 \text{ mg}/1000 \text{ mL} = \text{X mg}/5 \text{ mL}$$

$$\text{X} = 40 \text{ mg, answer}$$

Example 3:

A child weighing 12 kg is to receive 6 mg of phenytoin per kg of body weight daily as an anticonvulsant. How many milliliters of pediatric phenytoin suspension containing 30 mg per 5 mL should the child receive?

By setting up appropriate proportions, this type of a problem may be solved in two steps:

Step 1
Find the dose for the child.
6 mg/kg for a 12 kg patient. The patient should receive
$6 \times 12 = 72$ mg

Step 2
Find how many mL would contain that dose.
If 30 mg were contained in 5 mL, 72 mg would be contained in:
30 mg/5 mL = 72 mg/X mL
X = 12 mL, answer

PRACTICE PROBLEMS

1. A syrup contains the equivalent of 50 gr of active ingredient in each fluid ounce (480 minims) of the syrup. How many minims would provide the equivalent of 10 gr of the active ingredient?
2. A syrup contains the equivalent of 100 g of active ingredient in two fluid ounces of the syrup. How many minims would provide the equivalent of 5 g of the active ingredient?

3. If a pharmacist had two 1-liter stock bottles of each of the ingredients, how many times could the following prescription be filled?

   ℞

Aspirin syrup		10 mL
Simple syrup	ad	100 mL

   Sig. 5 mL as required

4. If a pharmacist had ten 1-liter stock bottles of each of the ingredients, how many times could the following prescription be filled?

   ℞

Codeine sulfate solution		5 mL
Simple syrup USP	ad	10 mL

   Sig. 5 mL as required for cough

5. How many mL of Elixir A would be taken in the initial dose of the prescription?

   ℞

Elixir A		
Elixir B	aa (of each)	10 mL
Suspension		50 mL

   Sig. 10 mL stat., then 5 mL t.i.d.

6. How many mL of verapamil solution would be taken in the initial dose of the prescription?

   ℞

Verapamil solution		
Simple syrup USP	aa (of each)	5 mL
Water		90 mL

   Sig. 15 mL stat., then 10 mL t.i.d.

7. How many grams of amiodarone should be used in compounding the following prescription?

   ℞

   Amiodarone
   Aromatic elixir aa q.s.
   Make a solution to contain 0.1 g/tsp
   Disp. 100 mL
   Sig. 5 mL daily

8. How many grams of calcium carbonate should be used in compounding the following prescription?

   ℞

   Calcium carbonate
   Simple syrup aa q.s.
   Make a solution to contain 0.05 g/tsp
   Disp. 250 mL
   Sig. 5 mL daily

9. How many mL of diazepam and aspartame are present in each 5-mL dose?

℞

Diazepam suspension		10.0 mL
Aspartame		0.2 g
Ethanol		1.0 mL
Purified water	ad	100.0 mL

Mix and make a suspension.
Sig. 5mL tid

10. How many mL of ephedrine sulfate and pseudoephedrine sulfate are present in each 10-mL dose?

℞

Ephedrine sulfate		5 mg
Pseudoephedrine sulfate		5 mg
Ethanol		1.0 mL
Purified water	ad	100.0 mL

Mix and make a suspension.
Sig. 10 mL daily

11. The equivalent of 32 gr of active ingredient is contained in each fluid ounce (480 minims) of a syrup. How many minims would provide the equivalent of 20 gr of the active ingredient?

12. If a pharmacist had four 1-liter stock bottles of each of the ingredients, how many times could the following prescription be filled?

℞

Actifid syrup		60 mL
Robitussin syrup	ad	120 mL

Sig. 5 mL as required for cough.

13. How many mL of Decadron® Elixir would be taken in the initial dose of the prescription?

℞

Decadron elixir		
Benadryl elixir	aa (of each)	20 mL
Triple sulfas suspension		80 mL

Sig. 10 mL stat., then 5 mL t.i.d.

14. How many grams of potassium thiocyanate should be used in compounding the following prescription?

℞

Potassium thiocyanate		
Aromatic elixir	aa	q.s.

Make a solution to contain 0.2 g/tsp
Disp. 150 mL
Sig. 5 mL in water daily

15. How many mL of paregoric and pectin are present in each 15-mL dose?

℞

Paregoric		15.0 mL
Pectin		0.5 g
Kaolin		20.0 g
Ethanol		1.0 mL
Purified water	ad	100.0 mL

Mix and make a suspension.
Sig. 15 mL p.r.n. for diarrhea.

16. ℞

Dihydrocodeinone gr 1/12 per tsp
Hydriodic acid syrup
Cherry syrup aa f℥-iii
Sig. Tsp. every 2 hr. for cough.
How many grains of dihydrocodeinone should be used in compounding the prescription?

17. A physician prescribes tetracycline suspension for a patient to be taken in doses of 2 teaspoonfuls 4 times a day for 4 days, and then 1 teaspoonful 4 times a day for 2 days. How many milliliters of the suspension should be dispensed to provide the quantity for the prescribed dosage regimen?
18. A medication order for theophylline oral suspension for a patient to be taken in doses of 1 teaspoonful 3 times a day for 5 days, and then 1 teaspoonful 2 times a day for 2 days. How many milliliters of the suspension should be dispensed to provide the quantity for the prescribed dosage regimen?
19. The pediatric dose of cefadroxil is 30 mg/kg/day. A child is receiving a daily dose of 2 teaspoonfuls of a pediatric cefadroxil suspension based on the body weight. If the child's weight is 18.3 lb, how many mg of the drug child is receiving in each dose?
20. A patient has been instructed to take 15 mL of Vistaril® (hydroxyzine pamoate) oral suspension every 6 hours for 4 doses daily. How many days will two 6-fluid-ounce bottles of the suspension last?
21. ℞

Codeine sulfate gr 1/6 per tsp
Cherry syrup q.s. f℥-ii
Sig. Tsp. every 2 hr. for cough.
How many grains of codeine sulfate should be used in compounding the prescription?

22. ℞

Omeprazole 0.5 g per tsp
Simple syrup q.s. f℥-iv
Sig. Tsp. every 6 hr.
How many grams of omeprazole should be used in compounding the prescription?

23. A physician prescribes theophylline suspension for a patient to be taken in doses of 2 teaspoonfuls 3 times a day for 3 days, and then 1 teaspoonful 3 times a day for 2 days. How many milliliters of the suspension should be dispensed to provide the quantity for the prescribed dosage regimen?
24. A doctor prescribes penicillin suspension for a patient to be taken in doses of 1 teaspoonful 4 times a day for 2 days, and then 1 teaspoonful 2 times a day for 2 days. How many milliliters of the suspension should be dispensed to provide the quantity for the prescribed dosage regimen?
25. A medication order for aminophylline oral suspension for a patient to be taken in doses of 2 teaspoonfuls 2 times a day for 5 days, and then 1 teaspoonful 2 times a day for 2 days. How many milliliters of the suspension should be dispensed to provide the quantity for the prescribed dosage regimen?
26. A medication order for $CaCO_3$ oral suspension for a patient is to be taken in doses of 3 teaspoonfuls 4 times a day for 2 days, and then 1 teaspoonful 2 times a day for 5 days. How many milliliters of the suspension should be dispensed to provide the quantity for the prescribed dosage regimen?
27. The pediatric dose of aspirin is 10 mg/kg/day. A child is receiving a daily dose of 2 teaspoonfuls of a pediatric aspirin suspension based on the body weight. If the child's weight is 22 lb, how many mg of the drug is the child receiving in each dose?
28. The pediatric dose of an antibiotic is 5 mg/kg/day. A child is receiving a daily dose of 1 teaspoonful of a pediatric cefadroxil suspension based on the body weight. If the child's weight is 15.4 lb, how many mg of the drug child is receiving in each dose?
29. A patient has been instructed to take 10 mL of tetracycline oral suspension every eight hours for three doses daily. How many days would one 4-fluid-ounce bottle of the suspension last?
30. A physician instructs a patient to take 5 mL of oral suspension every 4 hours for 5 doses daily. How many days would two 5-fluid-ounce bottles of the suspension last?
31. Codeine elixir contains 1 gr of codeine/fluid ounce. How much additional codeine should be added to 4 fluid ounces of the elixir so that each tsp will contain 15 mg of codeine?
32. How many mg each of noscapine and guaifenesin would be contained in each dose of the following prescription?

℞

Noscapine		0.60 g
Guaifenesin		4.80 g
Alcohol		15.00 mL
Cherry syrup	ad	100.00 mL

Sig. 5 mL t.i.d. p.r.n. cough.

33. If 2 fluid ounces of a cough syrup contain 20 gr of sodium citrate, how many milligrams are contained in 5 mL?

34. An elixir of ferrous sulfate contains 220 mg of ferrous sulfate in each 5 mL. If each mg of ferrous sulfate contains the equivalent of 0.2 mg of elemental iron, how many mg of elemental iron would be presented in each 5 mL of the elixir?
35. How many mL of Maalox suspension would be contained in each dose?

℞

Alurate elixir		10 mL
Maalox suspension	ad	60 mL
Sig. 5 mL t.i.d.		

36. How many milligrams of dextromethorphan should be used in filling the prescription?

℞

Dextromethorphan		15 mg/5 mL
Guaifenesin syrup	ad	f℥-viii
Sig. 5 mL q. 4h. p.r.n. cough.		

37. If a cough syrup contains 0.24 g of codeine in 120 mL, how many milligrams of codeine are contained in each teaspoonful dose?
38. If a potassium chloride elixir contains 40 milliequivalents of potassium ion in each 30 mL of elixir, how many mL will provide 15 milliequivalents of potassium ion to the patient?
39. The total dose of digoxin for rapid digitalization is 1 mg in two divided doses at intervals of 6 to 8 hours. How many milliliters of digoxin elixir containing 50 mcg/mL would provide this dose?
40. A physician ordered 1.5 mg of theophylline to be administered orally to a baby. How many milliliters of theophylline elixir containing 30 mg of theophylline per 10 mL should be used in filling the medication order?
41. Ticlopidine elixir contains 2 gr of ticlopidine/fluid ounce. How much additional ticlopidine should be added to 2 fluid ounces of the elixir so that each teaspoonful will contain 25 mg of ticlopidine?
42. Iodine elixir contains 1 g of iodine/fluid ounce. How much additional iodine should be added to 3 fluid ounces of the elixir so that each teaspoonful will contain 200 mg of iodine?
43. How many mg each of aspirin and caffeine would be contained in each dose of the following prescription?

℞

Aspirin		0.10 g
Caffeine		0.2 g
Alcohol		15.00 mL
Cherry Syrup	ad	100.00 mL
Sig. 5 mL t.i.d.		

44. How many mg each of benzoic acid and salicylic acid would be contained in each dose of the following prescription?

℞

Benzoic acid		0.30 g
Salicylic acid		0.5 g
Alcohol		15.00 mL
Water	ad	100.00 mL

Sig. 5 mL rub t.i.d.

45. If 2 fluid ounces of a solution contain 10 gr of quinapril HCl, how many milligrams are contained in 5 mL?
46. If 4 fluid ounces of a syrup contain 12 gr of pseudoephedrine, how many milligrams are contained in 1tsp?
47. A suspension of cadmium sulfate contains 100 mg of cadmium sulfate in each 5 mL. If each mg of cadmium sulfate contains the equivalent of 0.5 mg of elemental cadmium, how many mg of elemental iron would be presented in each 5 mL of the suspension?
48. A solution of sodium chloride contains 50 mg of sodium chloride in each 5 mL. If each mg of sodium chloride contains the equivalent of 0.5 mg of elemental sodium, how many mg of elemental sodium would be presented in each 5 mL of the solution?
49. How many mg of erythromycin would be contained in each dose?

℞

Erythromycin		10 mg
Potassium chloride suspension	ad	100 mL

Sig. 5 mL t.i.d.

50. How many mL of protamine sulfate suspension would be contained in each dose?

℞

Zinc susp		1mL
Protamine sulfate suspension	ad	100 mL

Sig. 5 mL t.i.d

51. How many milligrams of ubiquinone should be used in filling the prescription?

℞

Ubiquinone		30 mg/5 mL
Cherry syrup	ad	f℥-v

Sig. 5 mL b.i.d

52. How many milligrams of dextrose should be used in filling the prescription?

℞

Dextrose		12 mg/5 mL
Water	ad	f℥ -iii

53. If a suspension contains 0.10 g of barbiturate in 100 mL, how many milligrams of barbiturate are contained in each teaspoonful dose?
54. If a solution contains 0.5 g of nifedipine in 40 mL, how many milligrams of nifedipine are contained in each teaspoonful dose?
55. If a sodium nirtroprusside elixir contains 20 milliequivalents of sodium ion in each 20 mL of elixir, how many mL will provide 15 milliequivalents of sodium ion to the patient?
56. If a zinc chloride elixir contains 10 milliequivalents of zinc ion in each 60 mL of elixir, how many mL will provide 45 milliequivalents of zinc ion to the patient?
57. The total dose of methotrexate is 5 mg in two divided doses at intervals of 8 hours. How many milliliters of methotrexate elixir containing 100 mcg/mL would provide the total dose?
58. The total dose of prednisone is 12 mg in two divided doses at intervals of 8 hours. How many milliliters of prednisone elixir containing 5 mg/mL would provide this total dose?
59. A physician ordered 5 mg of cisapride to be administered orally to a patient. How many milliliters of cisapride elixir containing 20 mg of cisapride per 10 mL should be used in filling the medication order?
60. A physician ordered 1 mg of tamoxifen to be administered orally. How many milliliters of tamoxifen elixir containing 100 mg of tamoxifen per 50 mL should be used in filling the medication order?

LIQUID CALCULATIONS INVOLVING DILUTIONS AND CONCENTRATIONS

These types of calculations are encountered whenever there is a concentration or dilution change. When the solvent from a liquid medication is evaporated, its concentration is increased. On the other hand, when a liquid medication of a given strength is diluted, its strength will be reduced. For example, 10 mL of a solution containing 1 g of a substance has strength of 1:10 or 10% w/v. If this solution is diluted to 20 mL, i.e., the volume of the solution is doubled by adding 10 mL of solvent, the original strength will be reduced by one-half to 1:20 or 5% w/v.

To calculate the strength of a solution prepared by diluting a solution of known quantity and strength, an equation may be set up as follows:

$$C_1 \times V_1 = C_2 \times V_2$$

where,

C1 = Initial concentration
V1 = Initial volume
C2 = Final concentration after dilution
V2 = Final volume after dilution.

From this expression, strength (or final concentration) of the solution can be determined. To calculate the volume of solution of desired strength that can be made by diluting a known quantity of a solution, a similar expression may be used.

Example 1:

If 5 mL of a 10% w/v aqueous solution of genistein is diluted to 10 mL, what will be the final strength of genistein?

$$5\ (\text{mL}) \times 10(\%) = 10\ (\text{mL}) \times \text{X}(\%)$$

$$\text{X} = 5 \times 10/10 = 5\%\ \text{w/v, answer}$$

Example 2:

If a Tylenol® elixir containing 1.6% w/v APAP is evaporated to 90% of its volume, what is the strength of APAP in the remaining solution?

$$100\ (\text{mL}) \times 1.6(\%) = 90\ (\text{mL}) \times \text{X}(\%)$$

$$\text{X} = 160/90 = 1.78\%\ \text{w/v, answer}$$

Example 3:

How many milliliters of a 1:10 v/v solution of methyl salicylate in alcohol can be made from 100 mL of 2% v/v solution?

$$1{:}10 = 1/10 = 0.1\ \text{or}\ 10\%$$

$$100\ (\text{mL}) \times 2(\%) = \text{X}\ (\text{mL}) \times 10(\%)$$

$$\text{X} = 200/10 = 20\ \text{mL, answer}$$

PRACTICE PROBLEMS

1. If a phenasteride elixir containing 5% w/v phenasteride is evaporated to 70% of its volume, what is the strength of phenasteride in the remaining solution?
2. If an omeprazole elixir containing 7% w/v omeprazole is evaporated to 50% of its volume, what is the strength of omeprazole in the remaining solution?
3. If a prednisone elixir containing 9% w/v prednisone is evaporated to 30% of its volume, what is the strength of prednisone in the remaining solution?
4. If a lansoprasole elixir containing 11% w/v lansoprasole is evaporated to 15% of its volume, what is the strength of lansoprasole in the remaining solution?
5. If an albuterol elixir containing 2.5% w/v albuterol is evaporated to 85% of its volume, what is the strength of albuterol in the remaining solution?

6. If a lisinopril elixir containing 8% w/v lisinopril is evaporated to 40% of its volume, what is the strength of lisinopril in the remaining solution?
7. If a nabumetone elixir containing 12% w/v nabumetone is evaporated to 95% of its volume, what is the strength of nabumetone in the remaining solution?
8. If a paroxetine elixir containing 1% w/v paroxetine is evaporated to 10% of its volume, what is the strength of paroxetine in the remaining solution?
9. If a norfloxacin elixir containing 3% w/v norfloxacin is evaporated to 75% of its volume, what is the strength of norfloxacin in the remaining solution?
10. If a desipramine elixir containing 7% w/v desipramine is evaporated to 65% of its volume, what is the strength of desipramine in the remaining solution?
11. If 5 mL of a 20% w/v aqueous solution of furosemide is diluted to 10 mL, what will be the final strength of furosemide?
12. If a phenobarbital elixir containing 4% w/v phenobarbital is evaporated to 90% of its volume, what is the strength of phenobarbital in the remaining solution?
13. How many milliliters of a 1:20 v/v solution of methyl salicylate in alcohol can be made from 100 mL of 2% v/v solution?
14. If 5 mL of a 10% w/v aqueous solution of fluoxetine is diluted to 20 mL, what will be the final strength of fluoxetine?
15. If 15 mL of a 5% w/v aqueous solution of prochlorperazine is diluted to 45 mL, what will be the final strength of procholrperazine?
16. If 9 mL of a 10% w/v aqueous solution of estazolam is diluted to 25 mL, what will be the final strength of estazolam?
17. If 2 mL of a 2% w/v aqueous solution of minoxidil is diluted to 100 mL, what will be the final strength of minoxidil?
18. If 60 mL of a 10% w/v aqueous solution of salmeterol is diluted to 1200 mL, what will be the final strength of salmeterol?
19. If 17 mL of an 8% w/v aqueous solution of methylphenidate is diluted to 20 mL, what will be the final strength of methylphenidate?
20. If 14 mL of a 6% w/v aqueous solution of metoclopramide HCl is diluted to 38 mL, what will be the final strength of metoclopramide HCl?
21. How many milliliters of a 1:10 v/v solution of labetolol in alcohol can be made from 100 mL of 3% v/v solution?
22. How many milliliters of a 1:5 v/v solution of bromocriptine in alcohol can be made from 100 mL of 9% v/v solution?
23. How many milliliters of a 1:8 v/v solution of felodipine in alcohol can be made from 100 mL of 4% v/v solution?
24. How many milliliters of a 1:2 v/v solution of mefenamic acid in alcohol can be made from 100 mL of 7% v/v solution?
25. How many milliliters of a 1:6 v/v solution of dipyridamole in alcohol can be made from 100 mL of 8% v/v solution?
26. How many milliliters of a 1:9 v/v solution of norethindrone in alcohol can be made from 100 mL of 10% v/v solution?

27. How many milliliters of a 1:3 v/v solution of ketoprofen in alcohol can be made from 100 mL of 3% v/v solution?
28. How many milliliters of a 1:18 v/v solution of oxycodone in alcohol can be made from 100 mL of 8% v/v solution?
29. How many milliliters of a 1:33 v/v solution of chlorhexidine in alcohol can be made from 100 mL of 9% v/v solution?
30. How many milliliters of a 1:2 v/v solution of pravastatin in alcohol can be made from 100 mL of 6% v/v solution?

METHODS OF ALLIGATION

Alligation Medial

Alligation medial is a technique to determine the resultant concentration when two or more liquids of known concentrations are mixed. As an example, when 5 mL of 2% alcohol is mixed with 10 mL of 4% alcohol, we will know by the alligation medial method that we will obtain 15 mL of 3.33%. Essentially, the resulting strength is the "weighted average" of the percentage strengths of all the individual components used. Thus, the alligation medial is a method where the percentage strength of the mixture may be calculated by dividing the sum of the products of percentage strength of each constituent of the mixture multiplied by its corresponding quantity by the sum of the quantities mixed.

By the method of alligation medial, the percentage strength of a mixture may be calculated using three steps as shown below:

Step 1. Add the quantity of each component used in the mixture.
Step 2. Multiply the quantity of each component used in the mixture by its corresponding percentage strength, and add up the products.
Step 3. Divide the value obtained in Step 2 by the value obtained in Step 1.

The method of *alligation medial* may be best explained by the following examples:

Example 1:

What is the percentage of alcohol in the following mixture?

Alcohol 2% 5 mL
Alcohol 4% 10 mL

Step 1.

$5 + 10 = 15$ mL

Step 2.

$5 \times 2\% = 10$
$10 \times 4\% = \underline{40}$
50

Step 3.

$50/15 = 3.33\%$, answer

Example 2:

What is the percentage strength (v/v) of alcohol in a mixture of 10 mL of 10% v/v alcohol, 6 mL of 15% v/v alcohol, and 4 mL of 20% v/v alcohol?

Step 1.
$10 + 6 + 4 = 20$ mL
Step 2.
$10 \times 10 = 100$
$6 \times 15 = 90$
$4 \times 20 = 80$
270
Step 3.
$270/20 = 13.5\%$ v/v, answer.

Example 3:

What is the percentage of alcohol in the following prescription?

℞

Phenobarbital elixir	60 mL (15% alcohol)
Aromatic elixir	40 mL (22% alcohol)
Terpine hydrate elixir	50 mL (65% alcohol)
Purified water ad	250 mL
Sig. teaspoonful t.i.d.	

Step 1.
Total quantity is 250 mL.
Step 2.
Quantity of water used in the preparation $= 250 - (60 + 40 + 50) = 100$ mL
$60 \times 15 = 900$
$40 \times 22 = 880$
$50 \times 65 = 3250$
$100 \times 0 = 0$
5030
Step 3.
$5030/250 = 20.1\%$, answer

Alligation Alternate

Alligation alternate methods are very commonly employed to obtain a desired concentration of solution by mixing two or more liquids of known concentration. This is a very practical technique to obtain a medicine with prescribed concentration when two or more liquids of other concentrations are already available. By following this technique, we can obtain the prescribed medication without having actually to weigh the raw materials and mix them. Stated in other words, alligation alternate is a mathematical technique to obtain a desired concentration of a mixture when two or more solutions of known concentrations are available. The mixtures can be solutions or ointments. When the alligation alternate technique is used, it is important to remember that the desired solution's concentration has to be somewhere between the available concentrations. It cannot go beyond the boundaries of available concentrations.

The following steps may be used to find the proportional parts of each component to be used in a two-component mixture to obtain the desired strength:

1. Make three columns. In column 1, write the concentrations of the components to be mixed.
2. In column 2, write the desired percentage strength of the mixture to be prepared.
3. In column 3, write the difference in strength by reading diagonally (as illustrated in Example 1).
4. Find the relative proportions of the components (as illustrated in Example 1).

Example 1:

How many milliliters of oral calcium suspensions containing 300 mg per 5 mL and 1000 mg per 5 mL should be used in preparing 500 mL of a suspension containing 100 mg of calcium per mL?

300 mg per 5 mL is same as 60 mg/mL or 6%
1000 mg per 5 mL is same as 200 mg/mL or 20%
100 mg per mL is same as 10%

Column 1	Column 2	Column 3
6%		10 parts of 6% suspension
	10%	
20%		4 parts of 20% suspension
		----------
		14 parts in total

The quantities of each component to be used to obtain the specified quantity can be determined by the method of proportion as follows:

$$14/10 = 500/X$$

$$X = 357 \text{ mL of } 6\%$$

$$14/4 = 500/X$$

$$X = 143 \text{ mL of } 20\%, \text{ answer}$$

Example 2:

How many milliliters of a syrup having a specific gravity of 1.40 should be mixed with 1000 mL of a syrup having specific gravity of 1.2 to obtain a product having a specific gravity of 1.3?

Column 1 Column 2 Column 3

1.40 | | 0.1 parts

| 1.3 |

1.2 | | 0.1 parts

——–—

0.2 parts

The quantity of the syrup with the specific gravity of 1.2 is specified as 1000 mL. This equals 0.1 proportional parts. The proportional parts required for the syrup having a specific gravity of 1.40 is also 0.1. The quantity of the syrup with the specific gravity of 1.40 can be determined by the method of proportion as follows:

$$\frac{0.1}{0.1} = \frac{X}{1000\ \text{mL}}$$

X = 1000 mL of syrup with specific gravity of 1.40, answer

Example 3:

A physician writes for a medicated suspension to contain 50 mg of a steroid in 4 mL of normal saline solution (NSS). The pharmacist has on hand a 2.5% suspension of the steroid in NSS. How many milliliters of this and how many milliliters of NSS should be used in preparing the medication order?

If 50 mg are contained in 4 mL, the percentage strength may be calculated as follows:

$$0.05\ \text{g}/4\ \text{mL} = X\ \text{g}/100\ \text{mL}$$

$$X = 1.25\ \text{g}/100\ \text{mL or } 1.25\%$$

Column 1 Column 2 Column 3

2.5% | | 1.25 parts of 2.5% suspension

| 1.25 |

0% | | 1.25 parts of normal saline

Thus, a suspension of cortisone acetate of desired strength can be obtained by mixing equal parts (i.e., 1.25 parts or 2mL each) of 2.5% suspension and normal saline.

This may be confirmed by $C_1 \times V_1 = C_2 \times V_2$ method as follows:

$$4\ \text{mL} \times 1.25\% = X\ \text{mL} \times 2.5\%$$

$$X = (4 \times 1.25)/2.5$$

$$X = 2\ \text{mL}$$

Thus, 2 mL of 2.5% suspension and 2 mL of NSS may be mixed to contain 50 mg/4 mL, answer.

PRACTICE PROBLEMS

1. What is the percentage of alcohol in the following prescription?
   Tincture A 110 mL (35% alcohol)
   Tincture B 220 mL (25% alcohol)
   Tincture C 330 mL (20% alcohol)
   Sig. 5 mL for cough.
2. What is the percentage strength (v/v) of alcohol in a mixture of 20 mL of 12% v/v alcohol, 15 mL of 18% v/v alcohol, and 25 mL of 25% v/v alcohol?
3. What is the percentage strength (v/v) of alcohol in a mixture of 12 mL of 17% v/v alcohol, 10 mL of 50% v/v alcohol, and 500 mL of 33% v/v alcohol?
4. What is the percentage strength (v/v) of alcohol in a mixture of 32 mL of 35% v/v alcohol, 22 mL of 37% v/v alcohol, and 11 mL of 28% v/v alcohol?
5. How many milliliters of a 1:250 v/v solution of diazepam in alcohol can be made from 100 mL of 2.5% v/v solution?
6. How many milliliters of a 1:100 v/v solution of testosterone in alcohol can be made from 100 mL of 10% v/v solution?
7. How many milliliters of a 1:50 v/v solution of aspirin in alcohol can be made from 100 mL of 50% v/v solution?
8. If 100 mL of a Choledyl® elixir containing 10 mg/5 mL active ingredient (oxtriphylline) is diluted to 500 mL, what will be the final strength of oxtriphylline?
9. If 10 mL of an elixir containing 50 mg/10 mL active ingredient is diluted to 12 mL, what will be the final strength of active ingredient?
10. If 100 mL of an elixir containing 3 mg/5 mL theophylline is diluted to 150 mL, what will be the final strength of theophylline?
11. What is the percentage of alcohol in the following prescription?
    Chloroform spirit 110.0 mL (88% alcohol)
    Aromatic elixir 85.0 mL (22% alcohol)
    Terpin hydrate elixir 255.0 mL (40% alcohol)
    Sig. 5 mL for cough.
12. What is the percentage strength (v/v) of alcohol in a mixture of 200 mL of 12% v/v alcohol, 150 mL of 18% v/v alcohol, and 250 mL of 25% v/v alcohol?
13. How many milliliters of a 1:500 v/v solution of methyl salicylate in alcohol can be made from 100 mL of 5% v/v solution?
14. If 50 mL of a Choledyl® elixir containing 100 mg/5 mL active ingredient (oxtriphylline) is diluted to 250 mL, what will be the final strength of oxtriphylline?
15. How many milliliters of phenobarbital elixirs containing 20 mg per 5 mL and 30 mg per 5 mL should be used in preparing a liter of phenobarbital elixir containing 4.8 mg of phenobarbital per mL?

16. How many milliliters of methenamine mandelate oral suspensions containing 250 mg and 500 mg per 5 mL should be used in preparing a liter of a suspension containing 60 mg of methenamine mandelate per mL?
17. How many milliliters of griseofulvin oral suspensions containing 100 mg and 125 mg per mL should be used in preparing 100 mL of a suspension containing 12% of griseofulvin?
18. A physician order calls for a theophylline oral suspension to contain 100 mg of theophylline in 5 mL of aqueous vehicle. The pharmacist has on hand a 4.5% aqueous suspension of theophylline. How many mL of aqueous vehicle should be added to the preparation on hand in preparing the prescribed suspension?
19. What is the percentage of alcohol in the following prescription?

    Tincture iodine 10 mL (40% alcohol)
    Aromatic elixir 20 mL (56% alcohol)
    Terpin hydrate elixir 30 mL (4% alcohol)
    Sig. 5 mL for cough.
20. What is the percentage of alcohol in the following prescription?

    Spirit 120 mL (20% alcohol)
    Elixir A 432 mL (60% alcohol)
    Elixir B 345 mL (20% alcohol)
    Sig. 5 mL for cold
21. How many milliliters of ketamine elixirs containing 40 mg per 5 mL and 60 mg per 5 mL should be used in preparing a liter of ketamine elixir containing 9.6 mg of ketamine per mL?
22. How many milliliters of digoxin elixirs containing 10 mg per 5 mL and 15 mg per 5 mL should be used in preparing 500 mL of digoxin elixir containing 2.4 mg of digoxin per mL?
23. How many milliliters of ranitidine elixirs containing 12 mg per 10 mL and 32 mg per 5 mL should be used in preparing 3 liters of ranitidine elixir containing 5 mg of ranitidine per mL?
24. How many milliliters of calcium oral suspensions containing 300 mg and 450 mg per 5 mL should be used in preparing 2 liters of a suspension containing 70 mg of calcium per mL?
25. How many milliliters of barium oral suspensions containing 250 mg and 500 mg per 5 mL should be used in preparing 500 mL of a suspension containing 55 mg of barium per mL?
26. How many milliliters of calcitonin nasal solution containing 2.5 mg per 5 mL and 5 mg per mL should be used in preparing 200 mL of a solution containing 1 mg of calcitonin per mL?
27. How many milliliters of taxol suspensions containing 50 mg and 65 mg per mL should be used in preparing 50 mL of a suspension containing 6% of taxol?
28. How many milliliters of EDTA solution containing 150 mg and 175 mg per mL should be used in preparing 150 mL of a solution containing 16% of EDTA?

29. How many milliliters of methotraxate suspensions containing 260 mg and 400 mg per mL should be used in preparing 1000 mL of a suspension containing 30% of methotraxate?
30. A physician order calls for a ketoprofen oral suspension to contain 50 mg of ketoprofen in 5 mL of aqueous vehicle. The pharmacist has on hand a 1.5% aqueous suspension of ketoprofen. How many mL of aqueous vehicle should be added to the preparation on hand in preparing the prescribed suspension?

ANSWERS

Liquid Calculations Involving Proportions

1. 96 minims
2. 50 minims
3. 22 prescriptions
4. 2000
5. 1.43 mL
6. 0.75 mL
7. 2 g
8. 2.5 g
9. 0.5 mL diazepam suspension and 0.01 g of aspartame
10. 0.5 mg Ephedrine sulphate and 0.5 mg Pseudoephedrine sulphate
11. 300 minims
12. 66.67 or 66 in this case
13. 1.67 mL
14. 6 g
15. 2.25 mL of Paregonic and 0.075 g of pectin
16. 3 gr
17. 200 mL
18. 95 mL
19. 249.6 mg per day
20. 6 days
21. 2 gr
22. 12 g
23. 120 mL
24. 60 mL
25. 120 mL
26. 170 mL
27. 100 mg per day
28. 35 mg per day
29. 4 days
30. 12 days
31. 100 mg
32. Noscapine 0.03 g and Guaifensin 0.24 g
33. 108.6 mg
34. 44 mg
35. 4.17 mL
36. 720 mg
37. 10 mg
38. 11.25 mL
39. 10 mL
40. 0.5 mL
41. 40 mg
42. 600 mg
43. Aspirin 5 mg and caffeine 10 mg
44. Benzoic acid 15 mg and salicylic acid 25 mg
45. 54.17 mg
46. 32.5 mg
47. 50 mg
48. 25 mg
49. 0.5 mg
50. 4.95 mL
51. 900 mg
52. 216 mg
53. 5 mg
54. 62.5 mg
55. 15 mL
56. 270 mL
57. 50 mL

58. 2.4 mL
59. 2.5 mL
60. 0.5 mL
61. 10% w/v

Calculations Involving Dilutions and Concentration

1. 7.14% w/v
2. 14% w/v
3. 30% w/v
4. 73.3% w/v
5. 2.94% w/v
6. 20% w/v
7. 12.63% w/v
8. 10% w/v
9. 4% w/v
10. 10.77% w/v
11. 10% w/v
12. 4.44% w/v
13. 40 mL
14. 2.5% w/v
15. 1.67% w/v
16. 3.6% w/v
17. 0.04% w/v
18. 0.5% w/v
19. 6.8% w/v
20. 2.2% w/v
21. 30 mL
22. 45 mL
23. 32 mL
24. 14 mL
25. 48 mL
26. 90 mL
27. 9 mL
28. 144 mL
29. 300 mL
30. 12 mL

Alligation

1. 24.17%
2. 18.92%
3. 32.96%
4. 34.49%
5. 625 mL of a 1:250 v/v solution of diazepam in alcohol can be made from 100 mL of 2.5% v/v solution.
6. 1000 mL of a 1:100 v/v solution of testosterone in alcohol can be made from 100 mL of 10% v/v solution.
7. 2500 mL of a 1:50 v/v solution of aspirin in alcohol can be made from 100 mL of 50% v/v solution.
8. The final strength of choledyl elixir will be 0.04%.
9. The final strength of active ingredient will be 0.42% w/v.
10. The final strength of theophylline will be 0.04% w/v.
11. 48.33%
12. 18.92%
13. 2500 mL of a 1:500 v/v solution of methyl salicylate in alcohol can be made from 100 mL of 5% v/v solution.
14. The final strength of oxtriphylline will be 4 mg/mL or 0.4% w/v.
15. 600 mL of 0.4% and 400 mL of 0.6% are required to prepare the solution of required strength.
16. 800 mL of 5% and 200 mL of 10% are required to prepare the solution of required strength.
17. 20 mL of 10% and 80 mL of 12.5% are required to prepare the suspension of required strength.

18. 2.2 mL of 4.5% suspension and 2.8 mL of vehicle may be mixed to contain 100 mg/5 mL.
19. 27.33%
20. 39.26%
21. 600 mL of 0.8% and 400 mL of 1.2% are required to prepare the solution of required strength.
22. 300 mL of 0.2% and 200 mL of 0.3% are required to prepare the solution of required strength.
23. 807.7 mL of 0.12% and 2192.3 mL of 0.64% are required to prepare the solution of required strength.
24. 1333.3 mL of 6% and 666.7 mL of 9% are required to prepare the solution of required strength.
25. 450 mL of 5% and 50 mL of 10% are required to prepare the solution of required strength.
26. 177.8 mL of 0.05% and 22.2 mL of 0.5% are required to prepare the solution of required strength.
27. 16.7 mL of 5% and 33.3 mL of 6.5% are required to prepare the suspension of required strength.
28. 90 mL of 15% and 60 mL of 17.5% are required to prepare the solution of required strength.
29. 714.3 mL of 26% and 285.7 mL of 40% are required to prepare the suspension of required strength.
30. 3.3 mL of 1.5% suspension and 1.7 mL of vehicle may be mixed to obtain 50 mg/5 mL

8 Working with Solid Dosage Forms

Prescription and non-prescription drugs are most commonly filled in solid dosage form. Because tablets and capsules make up the bulk of solid dosage forms, their calculations are highlighted in this chapter. These dosage forms are usually available in several strengths. If a capsule or a tablet of higher strength is prescribed but unavailable, two capsules or tablets of one-half the strength may be dispensed. Thus, a pharmacist or a health care professional may need to administer one-half or some other portion of the tablet, for example, if 500 mg Keflex® capsules are prescribed, and the pharmacist or a nurse has only 250 mg capsules. In such a case, twice the total number of capsules required should be dispensed with the clear instructions to take two capsules to the patients.

Alternatively if a lower strength is prescribed and higher strength is available, the higher strength tablet may be split to provide the desired amount of drug. However, when the substitution of strengths is made it is important to remember that tablets that are not scored should not be broken. Another precaution to remember is when enteric-coated dosage forms are prescribed. Enteric-coated tablets are designed to resist the acidic environment in the stomach and release the medication in the small intestine. If such tablets are broken, their enteric properties may be lost. Therefore, do not break them. As a general rule, do not divide sustained/controlled release medications, as they may lose their controlled release properties. However, there may be some exceptions to this rule. For example, Calan® SR 240 tablets that are to be given once daily can be split to administer 120 mg (or 2 tablets) twice daily. Therefore, unless specifically suggested by the manufacturer, these tablets should not be crushed or broken.

Example 1:

If a prescription is received with the instructions of providing 650 mg of Tylenol® to a patient, and the pharmacist has 325 mg tablets, how many tablets should the patient be instructed to take?

Two tablets of Tylenol® 325 mg should be taken by the patient, answer

Example 2:

Zantac® is available in a strength of 300 mg. If a prescription is written for 150 mg bid for three weeks as directed, how many tablets should be dispensed?

One 300 mg tablet should be given for 1 day
For 21 days, 21 300 mg tablets should be dispensed, answer

Example 3:

℞
Ibuprofen 600 mg
#21
Sig. I tab tid, pc

Assume that the patient has a stock of Motrin®-IB (ibuprofen 200 mg) at home, and he decides to take them instead of getting the prescription filled by a pharmacist. How many Motrin tablets should the patient take in 1 day?

1 ibuprofen 600 mg = 3 Motrin-IB tablets
Therefore, the patient should take 9 Motrin®-IB tablets (3 × 3) every day, answer

PRACTICE PROBLEMS

1. A medication order reads "Give Tegretol 200 mg p. o. q. 12 hours for 2 weeks." Only 100 mg tablets are available. How many tablets should be dispensed?
2. Doctor's order reads "Neupogen 2.5 μg/lb." If the patient weighs 50 kg, how much you should give to the patient to provide the prescribed dose?
3. Doctor's order reads "Diflucan, iistat iqd for 10 days." How many Diflucan tablets should you give to the patient?
4. A medication order reads "100 mg Ultram twice a day for 2 months." If Ultram is available in a strength of 50 mg/tablet, how many tablets should be dispensed?
5. Vioxx is available as 7.5 mg/tablet. The doctor's order reads "1 tablet 3 times daily for 4 weeks." How many tablets should be dispensed?
6. A cortisone medication reads "One tablet twice a day for 3 days, then ½ tablet twice a day for 3 days, and ½ tablet once daily for 10-days" for 5mg/tablets cortisone. How many tablets should be dispensed?
7. A medication order reads "20 mg/famotidine per day for 3 weeks, then 20 mg per day every other day for a month." Only 10 mg/tablets are available. How many tablets should be dispensed for the 45-day treatment period?
8. Prednisone capsules 5 mg/capsule are available. A medication order reads "5 mg 3 times a day for 1 week, then 5 mg twice a day for the next week, and 5 mg once daily for another week and finally, 1 mg/day for 10 days." How many capsules should be dispensed?
9. A physician orders 600 mg ibuprofen 3 times a day after meal for 3 weeks. The patient has a bottle of 500 tablets ibuprofen 200 mg/tablets. The physician told him that he could use it instead of the prescribed ibuprofen. How many tablets of OTC ibuprofen will remain after the 3-week treatment period?

10. Doctor's order reads "Biaxin 500 mg twice a day for 10 days." How many 500 mg tablets should be dispensed?
11. If a prescription requires a stat dose of 0.375 mg of digoxin tablets, and the pharmacist has tablets of strength, 0.125 mg, how many of the lower strength digoxin tablets should the patient take?
12. ℞

    Cephalexin 500 mg
    Sig. i cap tid, 10 days
    If a pharmacist dispenses Keflex 250 mg capsules, what directions should be provided to the patient?
13. In the above problem, how many cephalexin 250 mg capsules should be dispensed totally?
14. Spironolactone tablets are available in 25 mg strength, but a drug order comes for 150 mg dose. How many tablets should be dispensed?
15. ℞

    Slow-K® 10 mEq
    #20
    Sig: 10 mEq bid

    If only 20 mEq tablets are available, how many 20 mEq tablets would you dispense as a pharmacist? Assume that the tablets can be split into halves.
16. ℞

    Phenobarbital gr i
    #42 tablets
    Sig: i tablet tid, finish all

    A pharmacist had 24 tablets of phenobarbital 32 mg. After notifying the physician, he dispensed those tablets to the patient. How long would that medication last?
17. ℞

    Synthroid® 100 mcg
    20 tablets
    Sig: i qd

    If a pharmacist dispensed Synthroid 25 mcg tablets, how many tablets would the patient take every day?
18. ℞

    V-Cillin® K
    800,000 units tid, 5 days

    If the available tablets have a strength of 250 mg, how many tablets should be dispensed? It is known that 1 mg of penicillin K = 1600 units.
19. Gantrisin® gr L
    #14

    Use as directed.

    500 milligram Gantrisin® tablets are available. How many tablets should be dispensed?

20. ℞
    Phenergan® tablets 12.5 mg
    Dispense 14 tablets
    Sig: ss qhs
    If the pharmacist dispensed 25 mg tablets of Phenergan,® how many tablets should the patient take at bedtime?
21. A medication order reads "Give Reglan 10 mg p.o.q. 12 hours for 2 weeks." Only 5 mg tablets are available. How many tablets should be dispensed?
22. Doctor's order reads "Neupogen 2.5 μg/lb." If the patient weighs 70 lb, how much should you give to the patient to provide the prescribed dose?
23. Doctor's order reads "Zithromax, iistat, iqd for 5 days." How many Zithromax tablets should you give to the patient?
24. A medication order reads "100 mg Ultram twice a day for 3 months." If Ultram is available in a strength of 50 mg/tablet, how many tablets should be dispensed?
25. Vioxx is available as 7.5 mg/tablet. The doctor's order reads "1 tablet 3 times daily for 2 weeks." How many tablets should be dispensed?
26. A 5-mg cortisone medication reads "One tablet twice a day for 3 days, then ½ tablet twice a day for 3 days, and ½ tablet once daily for 5 days." Only 5-mg/tablet cortisone is available. How many cortisone 5-mg tablets should be dispensed?
27. A medication order reads "20 mg/famotidine per day for 15 days, then 20 mg per day every other day for a month." Only 10 mg-tablets are available. How many tablets should be dispensed for the 45-day treatment period?
28. Dexamethasone is available in 2 mg-tablets. A medication order reads "2 mg 3 times a day for 1 week, then 2 mg twice a day for the next week, then 2 mg once/daily for another week and finally, 1 mg/day for 10 days." How many tablets should be dispensed?
29. A physician orders 800-mg ibuprofen 3 times a day after meals for 3 weeks. The patient has a bottle of 500 tablets ibuprofen 200 mg/tablets. The physician told him that he could use it instead of the prescribed ibuprofen. How many tablets of OTC ibuprofen will remain after the three-week treatment period?
30. Doctor's order reads "Biaxin 500 mg twice a day for 10 days." Only 250 mg-tablets are available. How many tablets should be dispensed and what instruction should be given to the patient?

ANSWERS

1. 56 tablets
2. 275 micrograms
3. 11 tablets (2 on first day, and 1 each on the remaining 9 days)
4. $4 \times 60 = 240$ tablets
5. $1 \times 3 \times 28 = 84$ tablets

6. 6 + 3 + 5 = 14 tablets
7. 21 + 15 = 36 tablets of 20 mg, or 72 tablets of 10 mg
8. 21 + 14 + 7 + 2 = 44 capsules
9. 9 × 21 = 189. Then 500–189 = 311
10. #20
11. 3 tablets of digoxin
12. Take 2 capsules 3 times a day for 10 days
13. 2 × 3 × 10 = 60
14. 150/25 = 6 tablets
15. #10
16. 2 tablets tid = 6 tablets daily of 32 mg strength. Then 24/6 = 4 days
17. 4 tablets
18. 500 mg tid for 5 days = 15 tablets of 500 mg, or 30 tablets of 250 mg
19. 3250/500 = 6.5 tablets. Therefore, 6.5 × 14 = 91 tablets
20. ¼ of the 25 mg tablet
21. 2 × 14 = 28 for 10 mg, or 56 for 5 mg.
22. 175 micrograms
23. 6 tablets
24. 4 × 90 = 360 tablets
25. 3 × 14 = 42 tablets
26. 11½ tablets
27. 1 × 15 + 15 = 30 tablets of 20-mg, or 60 tablets of 10-mg
28. 21 + 14 + 7 + 5 = 47 tablets
29. 12 per day × 21 = 252. Then 500 – 252 = 248 tablets left
30. 20 tablets of 500 mg, or 40 tablets of 250 mg.

9 Adjusting Isotonicity

When a dosage form is administered in an eye, ear, nose, or vascular site, it may cause a lot of discomfort to the patient if the preparations are not isotonic. Isotonicity refers to the equality of osmotic pressure exerted by the formulation and the body fluids such as plasma, blood, and tears. Whenever a solution is separated from a solvent by a "semipermeable membrane," the solvent passes across the membrane into the solution. This is the phenomenon of osmosis, which may be defined as the passage of solvent molecules across a semipermeable membrane against the concentration gradient. Osmosis can also occur when a concentrated solution is separated from a less concentrated solution by a semipermeable membrane. The pressure differential that develops across the membrane is called "osmotic pressure."

Body fluids have the same osmotic pressure as that of a 0.9% w/v sodium chloride solution. Solutions having the same osmotic pressure as that of 0.9% w/v NaCl solution are said to be *isotonic* with blood. Solutions with a higher osmotic pressure than body fluids are called *hypertonic* and those with a lower osmotic pressure are called *hypotonic*. When hypertonic solutions are administered in the eye or any delicate tissue, the water from the tissues is likely to be drawn in the formulation by osmosis. This results in shrinking of the tissues, which is a cause of a lot of irritation. Conversely, when hypotonic solutions are administered, the water from the formulations tends to get in the tissues or red blood cells that swell and lyse. The lysis of red blood cells causes the reddening of the associated tissues. When the drug formulation is administered as an isotonic preparation, there is no discomfort to the patient. Therefore it is important to learn the ways by which a preparation can be made isotonic.

DISSOCIATION (*i*) FACTOR CALCULATIONS

The dissociation factor is a measure of the extent of ionization of a chemical such as the drug substance. The extent of ionization is important because it affects the osmotic pressure. Osmotic pressure is a colligative property and is dependent on the number of particles of solute(s) in a solution. The total number of particles of a solute in a solution is the sum of the undissociated molecules and the number of ions into which the molecule dissociates. The number of ions, in turn, depends on the degree of ionization. Thus, a chemical that is highly ionized contributes a greater number of particles to the solution than the same amount of a poorly ionized chemical. When a chemical is a nonelectrolyte such as sucrose or urea, the concentration of the solution depends only on the number of molecules present. The values of the osmotic pressure and other colligative properties are approximately the same for equal concentrations of different nonelectrolyte solutions. The dissociation factor, symbolized by the letter *i*, can be calculated by dividing the total number of particles

TABLE 9.1
Number of Ions, Dissociation Factor (*i*), and Molecular Weight (M.W.) of Selected Compounds

	Ions	*i*	M. W.
Boric acid	1	1.0	61.8
Chlorobutanol	1	1.0	177
Dextrose, anhydrous	1	1.0	180
Dextrose, H_2O	1	1.0	198
Mannitol	1	1.0	182
Benzalkonium chloride	2	1.8	360
Cocaine HCl	2	1.8	340
Cromolyn sodium	2	1.8	512
Dipivefrin HCl	2	1.8	388
Ephedrine HCl	2	1.8	202
Epinephrine bitartrate	2	1.8	333
Eucatropine HCl	2	1.8	328
Homatropine HBr	2	1.8	356
Oxymetazoline HCl	2	1.8	297
Oxytetracycline HCl	2	1.8	497
Phenylephrine HCl	2	1.8	204
Procaine HCl	2	1.8	273
Scopolamine HBr.$3H_2O$	2	1.8	438
Silver nitrate	2	1.8	170
Sodium chloride	2	1.8	58
Sodium phosphate, monobasic, anhydrous	2	1.8	120
Sodium phosphate, monobasic.H_2O	2	1.8	138
Tetracaine HCl	2	1.8	301
Zinc sulfate.$7H_2O$	2	1.4	288
Atropine sulfate, H_2O	3	2.6	695
Ephedrine sulfate	3	2.6	429
Sodium phosphate, dibasic, anhydrous	3	2.6	142
Sodium phosphate, dibasic.$7H_2O$	3	2.6	268

(which include undissociated molecules and ions) in a solution by the number of particles before dissociation (Table 9.1).

$$\text{i.e., } i = \frac{\text{Total number of particles of solute in a solution after dissociation}}{\text{Number of particles before dissociation}}$$

Example 1:

What is the dissociation factor of KCl, having 60% dissociation in water?

Assume that we have 100 particles of KCl prior to dissociation. Upon 60% dissociation, 100 molecules of potassium chloride yield:

60 potassium ions
60 chloride ions
40 undissociated potassium chloride particles
160 total particles in solution
$i = 160/100 = 1.6$, answer

Example 2:

What is the dissociation factor of magnesium sulfate, having 80% dissociation in water?

Assume that we have 100 particles of magnesium sulfate prior to dissociation. Upon 80% dissociation, 100 molecules of magnesium sulfate yield:

80 magnesium ions
80 sulfate ions
20 undissociated magnesium sulfate particles
180 total particles in solution
$i = 180/100 = 1.8$, answer

Example 3:

What is the dissociation factor of sodium carbonate (Na_2CO_3), having 60% dissociation in water?

Assume that we have 100 particles of sodium carbonate prior to dissociation. Upon 60% dissociation, 100 molecules of sodium carbonate yield:

120 (60 × 2) sodium ions
60 carbonate ions
40 undissociated zinc chloride particles
220 total particles in solution
$i = 220/100 = 2.2$, answer

SODIUM CHLORIDE EQUIVALENTS OF DRUG SUBSTANCES

By definition, the sodium chloride equivalent of a chemical is the amount of sodium chloride (in grams or grains) that has the same osmotic pressure as that of 1 gram of the chemical. The sodium chloride equivalents are symbolized by the letter *E*. The E value can be found in standard tables that can be found in many pharmaceutics and calculations texts. In the present text, the E values are given in Table 9.2. The E value can also be calculated, if molecular weight and dissociation factor values are known, by the following equation:

$$E = \frac{\text{M.W. of NaCl}}{i \text{ value of NaCl}} \times \frac{i \text{ value of the chemical}}{\text{M.W. of the chemical}}$$

TABLE 9.2
Sodium Chloride Equivalents (E) and Freezing Point Depression ($\Delta T_f^{1\%}$) Values of Selected Compounds

Substance	E	$\Delta T_f^{1\%}$
Ammonium chloride	1.08	0.64
Apomorphine hydrochloride	0.14	0.08
Atropine sulfate	0.13	0.07
Boric acid	0.52	0.29
Chlorobutanol	0.18	0.14
Cocaine hydrochloride	0.16	0.09
Dextrose monohydrate	0.16	0.09
Ephedrine hydrochloride	0.30	0.18
Ephedrine sulfate	0.23	0.14
Epinephrine bitartrate	0.18	0.11
Epinephrine hydrochloride	0.29	0.17
Eucatropine hydrochloride	0.18	0.11
Fluorescein sodium	0.31	0.18
Glycerin	0.34	0.20
Naphazoline hydrochloride	0.27	0.16
Neomycin sulfate	0.11	0.06
Oxymetazoline	0.20	0.11
Phenol	0.35	0.20
Phenylephrine hydrochloride	0.32	0.18
Pilocarpine nitrate	0.22	0.14
Procaine hydrochloride	0.21	0.11
Scopolamine hydrobromide	0.12	0.07
Silver nitrate	0.33	0.19
Sodium chloride	1.00	0.58
Sulfacetamide sodium	0.23	0.14
Tetracaine hydrochloride	0.18	0.11
Zinc chloride	0.62	0.37
Zinc sulfate.$7H_2O$	0.15	0.09

Note: E = Sodium chloride equivalent, $\Delta T_f^{1\%}$ = Freezing point depression of 1% solution

Example 1:

Calculate the sodium chloride equivalent of a 1% solution of chlorbutanol. Chlorbutanol has a molecular weight of 177 and i of 1.

$$E = \frac{\text{M.W. of NaCl}}{i \text{ value of NaCl}} \times \frac{i \text{ value of chlorbutanol}}{\text{M.W. of chlorbutanol}}$$

$$E = \frac{58.5}{1.8} \times \frac{1}{177}$$

$$= \frac{58.5}{1.8 \times 177}$$

$= 0.18$, i.e., 1 g of chlorbutanol is equivalent to 0.18 g of NaCl.

Example 2:

Calculate the sodium chloride equivalent of a 1% homatropine hydrobromide.
Homatropine hydrobromide has a molecular weight of 358 and i of 1.8.

$$E = \frac{\text{M.W. of NaCl}}{i \text{ value of NaCl}} \times \frac{i \text{ value of homatropine hydrobromide}}{\text{M.W. of homatropine hydrobromide}}$$

$$E = \frac{58.5}{1.8} \times \frac{1.8}{358}$$

$$= \frac{105.3}{644.4}$$

$= 0.16$, i.e., 1 g of homatropine hydrobromide is equivalent to 0.16 g of NaCl.

Example 3:

Calculate the sodium chloride equivalent of a 1% silver nitrate.
Silver nitrate has a molecular weight of 170 and i of 1.8.

$$E = \frac{\text{M.w. of NaCl}}{i \text{ value of NaCl}} \times \frac{i \text{ value of silver nitrate}}{\text{M.W. of silver nitrate}}$$

$$E = \frac{58.5}{1.8} \times \frac{1.8}{170}$$

$$= \frac{105.3}{306}$$

$= 0.34$, i.e., 1 g of boric acid is equivalent to 0.34 g of NaCl.

ISOTONICITY ADJUSTMENTS BY SODIUM CHLORIDE EQUIVALENT METHOD

The sodium chloride equivalent method is the most commonly used method for isotonicity adjustments. The sodium chloride (in g) equivalent of any drug substance, as discussed earlier, is the amount of sodium chloride that is osmotically equivalent to 1 gram of the drug. The sodium chloride equivalents for selected compounds are listed in Table 9.2. Any hypotonic solution containing one or more drugs can be rendered isotonic by adding an appropriate quantity of sodium chloride. However, extreme care is needed for isotonicity adjustments of hypertonic solutions. If water is added to convert the hypertonic solution to an isotonic solution, the drug concentration will decrease and additional drug will have to be added. Therefore, isotonicity adjustments usually are done for hypotonic solutions. Following is a sample prescription that requires isotonic adjustments:

℞	
Naphazoline HCl	1%
Sodium chloride	q.s.
Purified water ad	100
Make isoton. sol.	
Sig. Gtt. i o.u.	

In the prescription above, 1% naphazoline is ordered. The sodium chloride equivalent of naphazoline hydrochloride is 0.27 (refer to Table 9.2). This means that 1% solution of naphazoline hydrochloride has the same osmotic pressure as that of 0.27% solution of sodium chloride. This solution is hypotonic. Addition of 0.63 g (i.e., 0.9 – 0.27 = 0.63) of sodium chloride per 100 mL of the 1% solution of naphazoline hydrochloride results in an isotonic solution.

To determine the amount of sodium chloride required to render a given solution isotonic, the following steps may be used:

Step 1. Determine how much sodium chloride is needed to render the formulation isotonic with body fluids (Remember isotonicity refers to 0.9% or 0.9 g/100 mL).

Step 2. Find the amount of sodium chloride represented by the ingredients in the prescription by multiplying the quantity of each ingredient by its E value. Add up all the values obtained. This is the total amount of sodium chloride represented by all the ingredients in the prescription.

Step 3. Subtract the total value obtained in Step 2 from the amount of sodium chloride required to render the formulation isotonic (i.e., the value obtained in Step 1). The value obtained in this step represents the amount of sodium chloride required to be added to render the solution isotonic.

Example 1:

Find the quantity of sodium chloride required in compounding the following prescription. The sodium chloride equivalent of sulfacetamide sodium is 0.16.

℞	
Sulfacetamide sodium	0.2
Sodium chloride	q.s.
Purified water ad	30.0
Make isoton. sol.	
Sig. One drop in each eye.	

Step 1. $(0.9/100) \times 30 = 0.27$ g
Step 2. $0.2 \times 0.23 = 0.046$ g
Step 3. $0.27 - 0.046$ or 0.224 g, answer

Example 2:

Find the quantity of sodium chloride to be used in compounding the following prescription. The sodium chloride equivalent of chlorbutanol is 0.18.

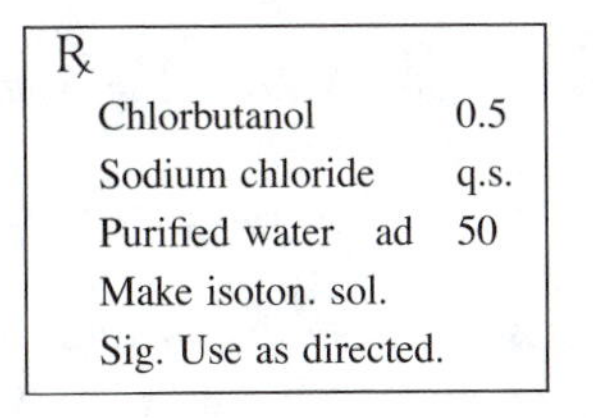
℞

Chlorbutanol	0.5
Sodium chloride	q.s.
Purified water ad	50
Make isoton. sol.	
Sig. Use as directed.	

Step 1. Sodium chloride needed to render the prescribed volume isotonic

$$(0.9/100) \times 50 = 0.45 \text{ g}$$

Step 2. $0.50 \times 0.18 = 0.09$ g
Step 3. g of sodium chloride needed to make the solution isotonic = $0.45 - 0.09 = 0.36$ g, answer

Example 3:

Find the quantity of sodium chloride to be used in compounding the following prescription. The values of sodium chloride equivalent of glycerine and scopolamine HBr are 0.34 and 0.12 respectively.

℞

Glycerine	1%
Scopolamine hydrobromide	0.5%
Sodium chloride	q.s.
Purified water ad	60.0
Make isoton. sol.	
Sig. Use in the eye.	

Step 1. Sodium chloride needed to render the prescribed volume isotonic

$$(0.9/100) \times 60 = 0.54 \text{ g}$$

Step 2. (a) Glycerine:

$$(1/100) \times 60 = 0.60$$

$$0.60 \times 0.34 = 0.204 \text{ g}$$

(b) Scopolamine HCl:

$$(0.5/100) \times 60 = 0.30$$

$$0.30 \times 0.12 = 0.036 \text{ g}$$

The total of sum of the weights (in g) of glycerine and scopolamine HCl multiplied by their E values, i.e., the total of (a) + (b) = 0.204 + 0.036 g = 0.24 g

Step 3. Sodium chloride to make the solution isotonic

$$0.54 - 0.24 = 0.30 \text{ g, answer}$$

If one desires to use a chemical other than sodium chloride, such as dextrose or boric acid, the quantity of that chemical can be calculated by dividing the value obtained in Step 3 (i.e., the amount of sodium chloride needed to render the solution isotonic with body fluids) by the E value of that chemical. A proportion can be set up which can be treated as Step 4 in addition to the three steps described earlier.

Example 1:

Find the quantity of boric acid (in grams) to be used in compounding the following prescription.

℞

Atropine sulfate	0.5%
Boric acid	q.s.
Purified water ad	30.0
Make isoton. sol.	
Sig. One drop in each eye.	

Step 1. (0.9/100) × 30 = 0.27 g

Step 2. (0.5/100) × 30 = 0.15 g
0.15 × 0.13 = 0.019 g

Step 3. 0.27 – 0.019 = 0.251

Step 4. From Step 3, 0.251 grams of sodium chloride are required to be added to make the preparation isotonic. But the prescription calls for boric acid as the tonicity agent. Boric acid has a E value of 0.52. This means that 1% boric acid is osmotically equivalent to 0.52% NaCl or 1 gram of boric acid is equivalent to 0.52 grams of NaCl.

$$\frac{1 \text{ g}}{0.52 \text{ g}} = \frac{x}{0.251 \text{ g}}$$

where x is grams of boric acid equivalent to 0.252 grams of sodium chloride.

Solving for x, we get: (0.251 × 1) ÷ 0.52 = 0.483 grams, answer

Example 2:

Find the quantity of boric acid (in grams) to be used in compounding the following prescription.

℞	
Chlorbutanol	0.1
Zinc sulfate	0.05
Boric acid	q.s.
Purified water ad	30.0
Make isoton. sol.	
Sig. Drop in eye.	

Sodium chloride equivalents are as follows:

Chlorbutanol = 0.18
Zinc sulfate = 0.15
Boric acid = 0.52

Step 1. $(0.9/100) \times 30 = 0.27$
Step 2. (a) Chlorbutanol:

$$0.1 \times 0.18 = 0.018 \text{ g}$$

(b) Zinc sulfate:

$$0.05 \times 0.15 = 0.0075 \text{ g}$$

$$a + b = 0.018 + 0.0075 \text{ g} = 0.0255 \text{ g}$$

Step 3. $0.27 - 0.0255 = 0.2445$ or 0.245 g
Step 4. From Step 3, 0.245 grams of sodium chloride is required to be added to make the preparation isotonic. But the prescription calls for boric acid as the tonicity agent. Boric acid has a *E* value of 0.52. To find the quantity of boric acid equivalent to 0.245 grams of sodium chloride, a proportion can be set up as follows:

$$\frac{1 \text{ g}}{0.52 \text{ g}} = \frac{x}{0.245 \text{ g}}$$

Solving for x, we get: $(0.245 \times 1) \div 0.52 = 0.471$ grams, answer

Example 3:

How many grams of dextrose should be used in compounding the prescription?

℞	
Sulfacetamide sodium	0.5
Chlorobutanol	0.25
Dextrose	q.s.
Rose water ad	50.0
Make isoton. sol.	
Sig. Nose drops.	

Sodium chloride equivalents are as follows:

Sulfacetamide sodium = 0.23
Chlorbutanol = 0.18
Dextrose = 0.16

Step 1. (0.9/100) × 50 = 0.45 g
Step 2. (a) Sulfacetamide sodium

$$0.50 \times 0.23 = 0.115 \text{ g}$$

(b) Chlorobutanol:

$$0.25 \times 0.18 = 0.045 \text{ g}$$

$$a + b = 0.115 + 0.045 \text{ g} = 0.16 \text{ g}$$

Step 3. 0.45 – 0.16 = 0.29 g

Step 4. $\dfrac{1 \text{ g}}{0.16 \text{ g}} = \dfrac{x}{0.29 \text{ g}}$

x = 1.812 g, answer

PRACTICE PROBLEMS

While solving these problems, refer to Table 9.1 and Table 9.2 as needed.

1. What is the dissociation factor of cocaine hydrochloride, having 20% dissociation in water?
2. What is the dissociation factor of homatropine hydrobromide, having 50% dissociation in water?
3. What is the dissociation factor of silver nitrate, having 90% dissociation in water?
4. What is the dissociation factor of atropine sulfate, having 40% dissociation in water?
5. What is the dissociation factor of ephedrine sulfate, having 70% dissociation in water?

6. What is the dissociation factor of phenylephrine hydrochloride, having 40% dissociation in water?
7. What is the dissociation factor of cromolyn sodium, having 30% dissociation in water?
8. What is the dissociation factor of dibasic sodium phosphate, having 60% dissociation in water?
9. What is the dissociation factor of scopolamine hydrobromide, having 30% dissociation in water?
10. What is the dissociation factor of oxytetracycline hydrochloride, having 40% dissociation in water?
11. Calculate the dissociation factor of pilocarpine hydrochloride, dissociating 80% in a certain concentration.
12. Calculate the *E* values of the following aqueous solutions at 1% concentration:
    (a) Chlorobutanol
    (b) Tetracaine hydrochloride
    (c) Ephedrine sulfate
13. How many grams of sodium chloride should be used in compounding the prescription?

    ℞

Procaine hydrochloride	1%
Sodium chloride	q.s.
Sterile water for injection ad	100

    Make isoton. sol.
    Sig. For injection.

14. How many grams of sodium chloride should be used in compounding the prescription?

    ℞

Cocaine hydrochloride	0.6
Eucatropine hydrochloride	0.6
Chlorobutanol	0.1
Sodium chloride	q.s.
Purified water ad	30.0

    Make isoton. sol.
    Sig. For the eye.

15. How many grams of boric acid should be used in compounding the following prescription?

    ℞

Zinc sulfate	0.06
Boric acid	q.s.
Purified water ad	30.0

    Make isoton. sol.
    Sig. Drop in eyes.

16. How many grams of sodium chloride should be used in compounding the prescription?

℞

Phenylephrine hydrochloride	1.0
Chlorobutanol	0.5
Sodium chloride	q.s.
Purified water ad	100.0

Make isoton. sol.
Sig. Use as directed.

17. How many grams of sodium chloride should be used in preparing the solution?

℞

Dextrose, monohydrate	2.0%
Sodium chloride	q.s.
Sterile water for injection ad	1000 mL

Label: Isotonic Dextrose and Saline Solution.

18. How many milliliters of a 5% solution of boric acid should be used in compounding the prescription?

℞

Oxymetazoline hydrochloride	2%
Boric Acid solution	q.s.
Purified water ad	15.0

Make isoton. sol.
Sig. For the nose, as decongestant.

19. How many grams of anhydrous dextrose should be used in preparing 1 liter of a ½% isotonic ephedrine sulfate nasal spray?
20. How many grams of boric acid should be used in compounding the prescription?

℞

Tetracaine hydrochloride	1.0
Boric acid	q.s.
Purified water ad	30.0

Make isoton. sol.
Sig. Eye drops.

21. Calculate the sodium chloride equivalent of a 5% solution of silver nitrate.
22. Calculate the sodium chloride equivalent of a 10% solution of procaine hydrochloride.
23. Calculate the sodium chloride equivalent of a 2% solution of scopolamine hydrobromide.
24. Calculate the sodium chloride equivalent of a 30% solution of hydrated sodium phosphate.

25. Calculate the sodium chloride equivalent of a 3% solution of cocaine hydrochloride.
26. Calculate the sodium chloride equivalent of a 25% solution of hydrated dextrose.
27. Calculate the sodium chloride equivalent of a 15% solution of mannitol.
28. Calculate the sodium chloride equivalent of a 5% solution of benzalkonium chloride.
29. Calculate the sodium chloride equivalent of a 10% solution of tetracaine hydrochloride.
30. Calculate the sodium chloride equivalent of a 10% solution of atropine sulfate.
31. How many grams of sodium chloride should be used in preparing 60 ml of a 2% isotonic pilocarpine nitrate ophthalmic solution?
32. How many grams of sodium chloride are needed in preparing 1 liter of a 2.5% isotonic silver nitrate solution?
33. How many milliliters of a 5% solution of sodium chloride are required to prepare 200 ml of a 3% isotonic atropine sulfate preparation?
34. How many milliliters of a 10% solution of sodium chloride should be used in compounding 50 ml of a 3% isotonic neomycin sulfate otic solution?
35. How many grams of dextrose monohydrate are needed in preparing 100 ml of a 5% isotonic hydrated zinc sulfate ophthalmic solution?
36. How many grams of boric acid should be used in preparing 1 liter of a 3% isotonic procaine hydrochloride topical solution?
37. How many milliliters of a 10% solution of dextrose monohydrate should be used in compounding 200 ml of a 5% isotonic chlorobutanol solution?
38. How many milliliters of a 20% solution of boric acid are required to compound 500 ml of a 2% isotonic naphazoline hydrochloride solution?
39. How many grams of sodium chloride should be used in preparing 1 liter of an isotonic solution containing 1% of epinephrine hydrochloride and 3% of neomycin sulfate?
40. How many grams of sodium chloride should be used in preparing 100 ml of an isotonic solution containing 1% of pilocarpine nitrate 2% of procaine hydrochloride?

ISOTONICITY ADJUSTMENTS BY CRYOSCOPIC METHOD

Isotonicity adjustments can also be made by the freezing point depression method. The normal freezing (or melting) point of a pure compound is the temperature at which the solid and the liquid phases are in equilibrium at a pressure of 1 atm. Pure water has a freezing point of 0°C. When solutes are added to water, its freezing point is lowered. The freezing point depression (or lowering) of a solvent is dependent *only* on the number of particles in the solution. Therefore, this is a colligative property. Blood plasma has a freezing point of –0.52°C (or freezing point depression of 0.52, i.e., 0 – [0.52]). If freezing point depression value of a chemical in certain concentration is known, one can calculate the concentration of that chemical required for isotonicity by setting a proportion as follows:

$$\frac{\text{Known percentage conc.}}{\text{Freezing point depression of the chemical at that concentration}} = \frac{X}{0.52°C}$$

where X = percentage concentration of the chemical required to be isotonic with blood plasma.

Since *freezing point depression* of a series of compounds at 1% concentration is readily available from standard references, the above expression can be represented as:

$$\frac{1\%\ \text{chemical}}{\Delta T_f^{1\%}\ \text{of the chemical}} = \frac{X}{\Delta T_f\ \text{of blood plasma } (0.52°C)}$$

where X = percentage concentration of the chemical required to be isotonic with blood plasma or tears.

Example 1:

1% boric acid solution has a freezing point depression of 0.29°C. What is the percentage concentration of boric acid required to make isotonic solution?

One can calculate the percentage concentration of boric acid by setting up the following proportion and solving for X:

$$\frac{1\%}{0.29} = \frac{X}{0.52}$$

$$X = (0.52 \times 1)/0.29$$

$$= 1.793 \text{ or } 1.79\% \text{ w/v}$$

It is known that 0.9% sodium chloride has the same osmotic pressure and the same freezing point depression of 0.52 as that of blood plasma, red blood cells, and tears. Drug solutions, which have a freezing point depression of 0.52, are, therefore, isotonic with blood. A list of freezing point depression values of selected compounds at 1% concentration is presented in Table 9.2. These ΔT_f values may be used to calculate the concentration of tonicity agents, such as sodium chloride or boric acid, needed to render a hypotonic drug solution isotonic with blood plasma. The following steps may be used to find the percentage concentration of NaCl required to render hypotonic drug solutions isotonic with blood plasma:

Step 1. Find the value of freezing point depression of the drug at 1% concentration, $\Delta T_f^{1\%}$, from Table 9.2.

Step 2. Subtract $\Delta T_f^{1\%}$ of the drug from the value of freezing point depression of 0.9% sodium chloride solution, i.e., 0.52. This difference may be symbolized as $\Delta T_f'$, which is the freezing point lowering needed for isotonicity.

Step 3. Since 0.9% sodium chloride has a freezing point depression of 0.52, one can calculate the percentage concentration of sodium chloride required to lower the difference in freezing points, i.e., the value obtained in Step 2, $\Delta T_f'$, by the method of proportion. The calculations involved in this method are explained best by the following examples.

Example 2:

Compound the following prescription.

℞	
Naphazoline HCl	1%
Sodium chloride	q.s.
Purified water ad	100
Make isoton. sol.	
Sig. One drop in each eye	

Step 1. Freezing point depression (ΔT_f) of 1% naphazoline solution (from Table 2) is 0.07.

Step 2. Find $\Delta T_f'$ by subtracting the ΔT_f value of 1% naphazoline hydrochloride from the ΔT_f of blood plasma, i.e., $0.52 - 0.07 = 0.45$. This means sufficient sodium chloride must be added to reduce the freezing point by an additional 0.45°C.

Step 3. Find the percentage concentration of sodium chloride required by setting up the proportion as follows:

$$\frac{0.9\%}{0.52} = \frac{X}{0.45}$$

In Table 9.2, it is observed that 1% solution of sodium chloride has a freezing point lowering of 0.58. Therefore, one can also express the proportion as:

$$\frac{1\%}{0.58} = \frac{X}{0.45}$$

Solving for X, we get: $(0.45/0.58) \times 1 = 0.78\%$

0.78% sodium chloride will render the above preparation isotonic. Thus, the isotonic solution will be prepared by dissolving 1.0 g of naphazoline hydrochloride and 0.78 g of sodium chloride in sufficient water to make 100 mL of solution.

Example 3:

Compound the following prescription.

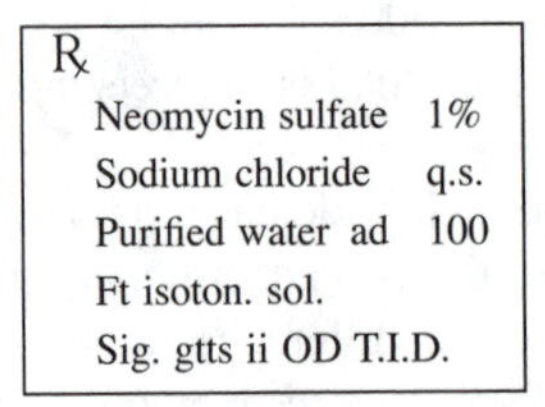

℞
Neomycin sulfate 1%
Sodium chloride q.s.
Purified water ad 100
Ft isoton. sol.
Sig. gtts ii OD T.I.D.

Step 1. Freezing point depression (ΔT_f) of 1% neomycin sulfate solution (from Table 9.2) is 0.06.

Step 2. Find $\Delta T_f'$ by subtracting the ΔT_f value of 1% neomycin sulfate from the ΔT_f of blood plasma, i.e., 0.52 − 0.06 = 0.48. This means, sufficient sodium chloride must be added to reduce the freezing point by an additional 0.48°C.

Step 3. Find the percentage concentration of sodium chloride required by setting up the proportion as follows:

$$\frac{0.9\%}{0.52} = \frac{X}{0.48}$$

or

$$\frac{1\%}{0.58} = \frac{X}{0.48}$$

Solving for X, we get: $(0.48/0.58) \times 1 = 0.83\%$

0.83% sodium chloride will render the above preparation isotonic. Thus, the isotonic solution will be prepared by dissolving 1.0 g of neomycin sulfate and 0.83 g of sodium chloride in sufficient water to make 100 mL of solution.

PRACTICE PROBLEMS

While solving these problems, refer to Table 9.1 and Table 9.2 as needed.

1. What is the percentage concentration of ammonium chloride required to make an isotonic solution?
2. What is the percentage concentration of chlorobutanol required to make an isotonic solution?
3. What is the percentage concentration of cocaine HCl required to make an isotonic solution?
4. What is the percentage concentration of dextrose monohydrate required to make an isotonic solution?

5. What is the percentage concentration of ephedrine HCl required to make an isotonic solution?
6. What is the percentage concentration of glycerin required to make an isotonic solution?
7. What is the percentage concentration of neomycin sulfate required to make an isotonic solution?
8. What is the percentage concentration of dextrose monohydrate required to make an isotonic solution?
9. What is the percentage concentration of oxymetazoline required to make an isotonic solution?
10. What is the percentage concentration of procaine HCl required to make an isotonic solution?
11. 1% boric acid solution has a freezing point depression of 0.29°C. What is the percentage concentration of boric acid required to make the solution isotonic?
12. 1% silver nitrate solution has a freezing point depression of 0.19°C. What is the percentage concentration of silver nitrate required to make an isotonic solution?
13. The freezing point of a 5% solution of eucatropine hydrochloride is –0.55°C. How many grams of eucatropine hydrochloride should be used in preparing 100 mL of an isotonic solution?
14. Determine if the following preparations are hypotonic, isotonic, or hypertonic:
    (a) A 7.5% atropine sulfate solution.
    (b) A parenteral infusion containing 20% (w/v) of dextrose.
    (c) A solution containing 2% ephedrine and 0.5% chlorobutanol.
    (d) A solution containing 2% phenol and 1% glycerin.
15. ℞

Ephedrine sulfate	1%
Sodium chloride	q.s.
Isotonic solution	40 mL

    Sig. gtt ii each nostril q6h
16. ℞

Phenylephrine HCl	0.5%
Boric acid	q.s.
Water qs	100 mL

    Sig. UD

    Make isotonic solution.
17. Adjust the isotonicity of the previous preparation using sodium chloride as the isotonic agent.
18. How much NaCl is required to render 100 mL of a 2% solution of epinephrine bitartarate isotonic with tears?
19. Freezing point depression of 1% pilocarpine nitrate is 0.14°C. Calculate the volume of an iso-osmotic solution produced by 1 gram of pilocarpine nitrate.

20. Freezing point depression of 1% fluorescein sodium is 0.18°C. Calculate the volume of an iso-osmotic solution produced by 1 gram of fluorescein.
21. How many milliliters of 10% scopolamine HBr are required to make a 200 ml isotonic solution?
22. How many milliliters of 5% silver nitrate are required to make a 250 ml isotonic solution?
23. How many milliliters of 5% sulfacetamide sodium are required to make a 100 ml isotonic solution?
24. How many milliliters of 20% tetracaine HCl are required to make a 60 ml isotonic solution?
25. How many milliliters of 5% zinc chloride are required to make a 150 ml isotonic solution?
26. How many milliliters of 10% zinc sulfate are required to make a 100 ml isotonic solution?
27. How many milliliters of 2.5% ammonium chloride are required to make a 100 ml isotonic solution?
28. How many milliliters of 5% chlorobutanol are required to make a 500 ml isotonic solution?
29. How many milliliters of 10% cocaine HCl are required to make a 500 ml isotonic solution?
30. How many milliliters of 5% ephedrine HCl are required to make a 250 ml isotonic solution?
31. How much sodium chloride is required to render 100 mL of a 1% solution of epinephrine HCl isotonic with tears?
32. How much sodium chloride is required to render 200 mL of a 2% solution of fluorescein sodium isotonic?
33. How much sodium chloride is required to render 500 mL of a 3% solution of naphazoline HCl isotonic?
34. How much sodium chloride is required to render 60 mL of a 5% solution of neomycin sulfate isotonic?
35. How much boric acid is required to render 200 mL of a 3% solution of procaine HCl isotonic?
36. How much boric acid is required to render 200 mL of a 5% solution of scopolamine HBr isotonic?
37. How much boric acid is required to render 60 mL of a 2% solution of silver nitrate isotonic?
38. How much boric acid is required to render 200 mL of a 3% solution of sulfacetamide sodium isotonic?
39. How much sodium chloride is required to render 200 mL of a solution isotonic? The solution contains 1% solution of pilocarpine nitrate and 2% of neomycin sulfate.
40. How much boric acid is required to render 200 mL of a solution isotonic? The solution contains 0.5% solution of scopolamine HBr and 1% of zinc chloride.

ANSWERS

Dissociation factor, sodium chloride equivalents of drug substances, and isotonicity adjustments by sodium chloride equivalent method:

1. 1.2
2. 1.5
3. 1.9
4. 1.8
5. 2.4
6. 1.4
7. 1.3
8. 2.2
9. 1.3
10. 1.4
11. 1.8
12. see below
    a. 0.18
    b. 0.19
    c. 0.20
13. 0.69 g
14. 0.048 g
15. 0.5 g
16. 0.49
17. 5.8 g
18. 2.88 mL of 5% boric acid solution and qs with water to 15 mL
19. 49.06 g
20. 0.173 g
21. 0.34
22. 0.21
23. 0.13
24. 0.42
25. 0.17
26. 0.16
27. 0.18
28. 0.16
29. 0.19
30. 0.12
31. 0.28
32. 0.75 g
33. 20.4 mL
34. 2.9 mL
35. 0.94 g
36. 5.19 g
37. 0 mL
38. 17.3 mL
39. 2.8 g
40. 0.26 g

Isotonicity adjustments by cryoscopic method:

1. 0.81%
2. 3.71%
3. 5.78%
4. 5.78%
5. 2.89%
6. 2.60%
7. 8.67%
8. 5.78%
9. 4.73%
10. 4.73%
11. 1.79%
12. 2.74%
13. 4.73%
14. See below
    a. Hypotonic
    b. Hypertonic
    c. Hypotonic
    d. Hypertonic
15. NaCl needed = 263 mg
16. Boric acid needed = 1.48 g
17. 0.74 g
18. 0.52 by cryoscopic method, and 0.54 g by E method
19. 26.9 mL
20. 34.6 mL
21. 149 mL

22. 137 mL
23. 74 mL
24. 14 mL
25. 42 mL
26. 58 mL
27. 33 mL
28. 371 mL
29. 289 mL
30. 144 mL
31. 0.61 g
32. 0.55 g
33. 0.35 g
34. 0.23 g
35. 1.31 g
36. 1.17 g
37. 0.29 g
38. 0.69 g
39. 0.90 g
40. 0.06. g

10 Working with pH and Buffers

pH CALCULATIONS

Maintenance of an appropriate pH is important for certain solutions and suspensions. This is because many drug substances are known to have greater solubility or stability at a certain known pH. Moreover, certain preparations are known to cause discomfort at certain pH values. For example, ear preparations cause discomfort when the solution pH is less than 4. The pH is defined as the as the *negative logarithm of the hydrogen ion concentration or logarithm of the reciprocal of the hydrogen ion concentration*. Since values of hydrogen ion concentration are very small, they are expressed in exponential notation as pH.

$$pH = -\log\left[H^+\right] \text{ or } \log 1/\left[H^+\right]$$

However, a bare proton does not exist by itself in water but is hydrated. Therefore, the above expression can also be written as:

$$pH = -\log\left[H_3O^+\right]$$

where $[H^+]$ or $[H_3O^+]$ indicates the molar concentration of hydrogen or hydronium ion. This expression may also be represented as:

$$\left[H^+\right] \text{ or } \left[H_3O^+\right] = 10^{-pH}$$

The pH values of topical dosage forms are adjusted for various reasons, including minimization of discomfort, maintenance of chemical stability, and improvement of therapeutic response.

CONVERSION OF HYDROGEN ION CONCENTRATION TO pH

Example 1:

What is the pH value of a solution whose hydrogen ion concentration is 2.88×10^{-3} moles per liter?

Solution:

$$\begin{aligned} pH &= -\log\left[H^+\right] \\ &= -\log\ 2.88 \times 10^{-3} \\ &= 2.54 \end{aligned}$$

Example 2:

What is the pH of a 7.93×10^{-4} molar solution of a strong acid?

Solution:

$$\begin{aligned} pH &= -\log\left[H^+\right] \\ &= -\log\left(7.93 \times 10^{-4}\right) \\ &= 3.1 \end{aligned}$$

Example 3:

What is the pH of a 0.00379 *M* solution of HNO_3?

Solution:

$$\begin{aligned} pH &= -\log\left[H^+\right] \\ &= -\log(0.00379) \\ &= 2.42 \end{aligned}$$

CONVERSION OF pH TO HYDROGEN ION CONCENTRATION

Example 1:

The pH of a Gifford ophthalmic solution is 6.2. What is the hydrogen ion concentration of this solution?

Solution:

$$pH = -\log\left[H^+\right]$$

$$\log\left[H^+\right] = -6.2$$

$$\begin{aligned} \left[H^+\right] &= \text{antilog of } -6.2 \\ &= 6.3 \times 10^{-7} \end{aligned}$$

It can also be solved as,

$$H^+ = 10^{-pH}$$
$$= 10^{-6.2}$$
$$= 6.3 \times 10^{-7}\ M$$

Example 2:

The pH of Palitz ophthalmic buffer solution is 8.2. What is the hydrogen ion concentration of this solution?

Solution:

$$H^+ = 10^{-pH}$$
$$= 10^{-8.2}$$
$$= 6 \times 10^{-9}\ M$$

Example 3:

The pH of a Sorensen modified phosphate buffer solution is 5.9. Calculate the hydrogen ion concentration of this solution?

Solution:

$$H^+ = 10^{-pH}$$
$$= 10^{-5.9}$$
$$= 1.26 \times 10^{-6}\ M$$

PRACTICE PROBLEMS

1. The hydrogen ion concentration of a solution is 0.00024 moles /L. What is the pH value of this solution?
2. The hydrogen ion concentration of a solution is 6×10^{-7} moles/L. What is the pH value of this solution?
3. The hydrogen ion concentration of a solution is 0.000038 moles/L. What is the pH value of this solution?
4. Convert the hydroxyl ion concentration, 0.00915 *M* to pH.
5. The pH of a Feldman ophthalmic buffer solution is 0.5. Calculate the hydrogen ion concentration in this solution.
6. The pH of 0.5% solution of barbital is 4.73. Calculate the hydrogen ion concentration in the solution.

7. The pH of 0.3 aqueous solution of codeine base at 25°C is 10. What is the hydrogen ion concentration in this solution?
8. The pH of an Atkin and Pankin ophthalmic buffer solution is 7.6. What is the hydrogen ion concentration in this solution?
9. Calculate the hydrogen ion concentration, if the pH of different Atkins and Pantin buffer solutions are:
   a. 7.6
   b. 8.5
   c. 8.8
   d. 9.4
10. Calculate the hydrogen ion concentrations of different Feldman ophthalmic buffer solutions having the following pH values:
    a. 6.0
    b. 6.9
    c. 7.1
    d. 7.4
11. What are the pH values of the following Gifford buffer solutions having the hydrogen ion concentration values of ______?
    a. 0.000001
    b. 6.31×10^{-7} *M*
    c. 1.26×10^{-7} *M*
    d. 6.31×10^{-8} *M*
    e. 3.16×10^{-8} *M*
12. Calculate the pH values of different Palitzsch ophthalmic buffer solutions having the following hydrogen ion concentration values:
    a. 1.259×10^{-8} moles/L
    b. 6.31×10^{-9} moles/L
    c. 2.51×10^{-9} moles/L
    d. 7.94×10^{-10} moles/L
    e. 5.25×10^{-10} moles/L
13. A phosphate buffer solution has pH 7.4. What is the hydronium ion concentration in this solution?
14. What is the hydroxyl ion concentration of the above solution?
15. Calculate the pH of 0.1 *N* solution of hydrochloric acid.

BUFFER CALCULATIONS

Buffer solutions are required to maintain the pH of a solution constant. Buffers contain mixtures of weak acids and their salts, or mixtures of weak bases and their conjugate acids. The ability to resist changes in pH is called buffer action or buffer efficiency. Some common buffer systems used in pharmaceutical dosage forms include mixtures of boric acid and sodium borate, acetic acid and sodium acetate, and sodium acid phosphate and disodium phosphate.

The concentration of buffer components needed to maintain a solution at the desired or required pH may be calculated by using buffer equations derived by Henderson–Hasselbalch as follows:

For weak acids
$$pH = pK_a + \log \frac{[\text{salt}]}{[\text{acid}]}$$
For weak bases
$$pH = pK_a + \log \frac{[\text{base}]}{[\text{salt}]}$$

where pK_a is the negative logarithm of the acid dissociation constant or acidity constant, K_a:

$$pK_a = -\log K_a \left(\text{or } K_a = 10^{-pK_a}\right)$$

Similarly, pK_b is the logarithm of the reciprocal of the basicity constant, Kb.

$$\therefore pK_b = -\log K_b \left(\text{or } K_b = 10^{-pK_b}\right)$$

Using appropriate buffer equations, one can calculate: (a) the pH value of a buffer system when pK and molar ratio (or concentration) of buffer components is known, and (b) the molar ratio of buffer components required to prepare a buffer with desired pH value.

The ion product (also referred to as "autoprotolysis constant") of water is symbolized by pK_w, which is equal to a value of 14. The values of pK_a and pK_b or pH and pOH are related to pK_w as follows:

$$pK_w = pK_a + pK_b = 14$$

$$pK_w = pH + pOH = 14$$

pH VALUE OF A BUFFER

Example 1:

What is the pH of a solution containing 0.2 mole of ephedrine and 0.002 mole of ephedrine hydrochloride per liter of solution? pK_a of ephedrine is 9.36 at 25°C.

Solution: Ephedrine is a weakly basic drug. Therefore one can use:

$$pH = pK_a + \log[\text{base}]/[\text{salt}]$$

$$= 9.36 + \log[0.2]/[0.002]$$

$$= 9.36 + \log 100$$

$$= 9.36 + 2 = 11.36, \text{ answer}$$

Example 2:

What is pH of Balitzsch buffer solution prepared with 0.1 *M* boric acid solution and 0.025 *M* sodium borate solution? The pK_a for boric acid is 9.24.

Solution: By applying the buffer equation for weak acid:

$$pH = pK_a + \log\frac{salt}{acid}$$

$$= 9.24 + \log\frac{0.025}{0.1}$$

$$= 9.24 + (\log 0.025 - \log 0.1)$$

$$= 9.24 - 0.6 = 8.64$$

Example 3:

What is pH of a buffer solution prepared with 0.3 *M* ammonium hydroxide and 0.3 *M* ammonium chloride solutions? The K_b for ammonium hydroxide is 0.000018 at 25°C.

Solution: By applying the buffer equation for weak base:

$$pH = pK_w - pK_b + \log\frac{base}{salt}$$

$$\because K_w \textit{ for water at } 25 \textit{ degree} = 10^{-14} \qquad \therefore pK_w = 14$$

$$K_b = 1.8 \times 10^{-5}$$

$$\because pK_b = -\log K_b$$

$$\therefore \log K_b = \log 1.8 + \log 10^{-5}$$

$$= \log 10^5 - \log 1.8 = 5 - 0.255 = 4.74$$

$$pH = 14 - 4.74 + \log\frac{0.3}{0.3}$$

$$pH = 9.26 - \log 1 = 9.26 - 0 = 9.26$$

MOLAR RATIO OF BUFFER COMPONENTS

Using the buffer (Henderson–Hasselbalch) equation, one can calculate the molar ratio of buffer components needed to prepare a buffer of desired pH. This is explained in the following examples.

Example 1:

What is the molar ratio of salt/acid required to prepare an acetic acid buffer of pH 4.2, using the pK_a of acetic acid of 4.76 at 25°C?

Solution: Using the buffer equation for weak acid:

$$pH = pK_a + \log\frac{salt}{acid}$$

$$4.2 = 4.76 + \log\frac{salt}{acid}$$

$$4.2 - 4.76 = \log\frac{salt}{acid}$$

$$\log\frac{salt}{acid} = -0.56$$

$$\frac{salt}{acid} = antilog\ of\ -0.56$$

$$\frac{\text{salt}}{\text{acid}} = \frac{0.275}{1} \text{ or } \frac{27.5}{100}$$

Example 2:

What is the molar ratio of salt/acid required to prepare a citric acid buffer having pH 5, using the pK_a of citric acid of 5.4 at 25°C?

Solution: Using the buffer equation for weak acid:

$$pH = pK_a + \log\frac{salt}{acid}$$

$$5 = 5.4 + \log\frac{salt}{acid}$$

$$5 - 5.4 = \log\frac{salt}{acid}$$

$$\log\frac{salt}{acid} = -0.4$$

$$\frac{salt}{acid} = antilog\ of -0.4$$

$$\frac{\text{salt}}{\text{acid}} = \frac{0.398}{1} \text{ or } \frac{39.8}{100}$$

Example 3:

What is the molar ratio of base/salt required to prepare ammonia buffer having the pH of 7.8, assuming that the pK_a of ammonium hydroxide is 9.24 at 25°C.

Solution: Using the buffer equation for weak base:

$$pH = pK_w - pK_b + \log\frac{base}{salt}$$

$$7.8 = 14 - 9.24 + \log\frac{base}{salt}$$

$$\log\frac{base}{salt} = 7.8 - 4.76$$

$$\frac{base}{salt} = antilog\ of\ 3.04$$

$$\frac{base}{salt} = \frac{1096.5}{1}\ or\ \frac{109{,}650}{100}$$

PRACTICE PROBLEMS

1. What is the pH of a buffer solution containing 0.04 *M* sodium maleate solution and 0.8 *M* maleic acid solution in one-liter, assuming that the dissociation constant of maleic acid is 5.5×10^{-7} at 25°C?
2. What is the pH of a buffer solution containing 0.08M formic acid solution and 0.2 *M* sodium formate solution in one-liter, assuming that the pK_a of formic acid is 3.75 at 25°C?
3. What is the pH of a buffer solution containing 0.2 *M* ammonium hydroxide solution and 0.04 *M* ammonium chloride solution in one-liter, using the Ka of ammonia as 5.75×10^{-10} at 25°C?
4. What is the pH of a solution containing 0.05 *M* atropine sulfate solution and 0.5 *M* atropine solution in one-liter, using the K_b of atropine as 4.47×10^{-5} at 15°C?
5. What is the pH of a solution containing 0.8 *M* morphine and 0.025 *M* morphine sulfate solution in one-liter, using the pK_a of morphine as 7.87 at 25°C?
6. What is the pH of a solution containing 0.65 *M* pilocarpine solution and 0.65 *M* pilocarpine sulfate solution in one-liter, using the K_b of pilocarpine as 7.0×10^{-8} at 25°C?
7. What is the pH of a solution containing 0.09 *M* pseudotropine solution and 0.3 *M* pseudotropine sulfate solution in one-liter, using the K_a of pseudotropine is 6.2×10^{-11} at 25°C?
8. What is the molar ratio of salt/acid needed to prepare a citric acid buffer having the pH 5.2? The pK_a of citric acid is 4.78 at 25°C?

9. What is the molar ratio of salt/acid needed to prepare citric acid buffer having the pH 2.8, using a pK_a of citric acid as 3.15 at 25°C?
10. What is the molar ratio of salt/acid needed to prepare oxalic acid buffer having the pH 5.8, using a pK_a of oxalic acid of 1.19 at 25°C?
11. What is the pH of a liter buffer solution containing 0.6 *M* sodium acetate and 0.15 *M* acetic acid? The pk_a for acetic acid equals 4.76 at 25°C.
12. What is the pH of a liter buffer solution containing 0.2 *M* acetic acid and 0.7 *M* potassium acetate? The K_a of acetic acid equals 1.75×10^{-5} at 25°C.
13. What is pH of a liter buffer solution containing 0.4 *M* benzoic acid and 0.045 *M* sodium benzoate? The pK_a for benzoic acid equals 4.2 at 25°C.
14. What is pH of a liter buffer solution containing 0.6 *M* benzoic acid and 0.07 *M* sodium benzoate? The dissociation constant (K_a) for benzoic acid at 25°C is 6.3×10^{-5}.
15. What is the pH of a liter buffer solution containing 0.5 *M* boric acid and 0.25 sodium borate per liter? The pK_a of boric acid is 9.24 at 25°C.
16. What is the pH of a liter buffer solution containing 0.7 *M* boric acid and 0.5 *M* sodium borate? The dissociation constant for boric acid is 5.8×10^{-10} at 25°C.
17. What is the pH of a liter citrate buffer solution containing 0.3M citric acid and 0.2M potassium citrate? The dissociation constant of citric acid is 4.0×10^{-6} at 25°C.
18. What is the pH of a buffer solution containing 0.005 *M* oxalic acid and 0.05 *M* potassium oxalate solution in one-liter? The dissociation constant of oxalic acid is 6.5×10^{-2} at 25°C.
19. What is the pH of a buffer solution containing 0.06 *M* oxalic acid solution and 0.4 *M* sodium oxalate solution in one-liter, assuming the dissociation constant of oxalic acid is 6.5×10^{-2}.
20. What is the pH of a buffer solution containing 2 *M* potassium oxalate solution and 0.02 *M* oxalic solution in one-liter, assuming the pK_a of oxalic acid is 4.21 at 25°C?
21. What is the molar ratio of base/salt required to prepare a buffer of ammonium hydroxide and ammonium chloride having the pH 7.8, using a pK_b of ammonium as 4.76 at 25°C?
22. What percentage of atropine base exists as unionized (base form) in ophthalmic drops buffered at pH 6.8, using a pK_b of atropine of 4.35 at 25°C?
23. What percentage of codeine base remains unionized in cough sedative syrup buffered at pH 7.0, using a pK_a of codeine of 7.95 at 25°C?
24. What is the molar ratio of base/salt in colchicine base solution buffered to pH 1.8, using a K_a of colchicine of 2.23×10^{-2} at 25°C?
25. What is the molar ratio of salt/base required to adjust the pH to 8.5 using ammonium hydroxide-ammonium chloride buffer, using K_b of ammonium hydroxide of 1.77×10^{-5} at 25°C?
26. What percentage of codeine base is expected to exist in the unionized form in cough sedative syrup buffered at pH 6.5, using a pK_a of codeine of 7.95 at 25°C?

27. What is the pH of a buffer solution containing 0.095 *M* acetic acid and 0.6 *M* sodium acetate? The dissociation constant of acetic acid is 1.75×10^{-5} at 25°C.
28. What is the molar ratio of salt/base required to prepare a buffer of ephedrine and ephedrine hydrochloride having pH 8.8? The pK_a of ephedrine is 9.36 at 25°C.
29. What is the molar ratio of boric acid/sodium borate required to prepare boric acid ophthalmic solution of pH 6.5? The pK_a of boric acid is 9.24.
30. What is the molar ratio of ammonium chloride/ammonium hydroxide required to prepare ammonia buffer of pH 9.25? The Kb of ammonium hydroxide is 1.8×10^{-5} at 25°C.

ANSWERS

pH

1. 3.62
2. 6.22
3. 4.42
4. 11.96
5. 0.32
6. 1.86×10^{-5}
7. 1×10^{-10}
8. 2.5×10^{-8}
9. (a) 2.51×10^{-8};
   (b) 3.16×10^{-9};
   (c) 1.58×10^{-9};
   (d) 3.98×10^{-10}
10. (a) 1×10^{-6};
    (b) 1.26×10^{-7};
    (c) 7.94×10^{-8};
    (d) 3.98×10^{-8}
11. (a) 6;
    (b) 6.2;
    (c) 6.9;
    (d) 7.2;
    (e) 7.5
12. (a) 7.9;
    (b) 8.2;
    (c) 8.6;
    (d) 9.1;
    (e) 7.28
13. 3.98×10^{-8}
14. 2×10^{-7}
15. 1

Buffers

1. 4.96
2. 4.15
3. 9.94
4. 10.65
5. 9.38
6. 6.85
7. 9.69
8. 2.63:1 or 263:100
9. 0.45:1 or 45:100
10. 40738:1
11. 5.36
12. 5.30
13. 3.25
14. 3.27
15. 8.94
16. 9.09
17. 5.22
18. 2.19
19. 2.01
20. 6.21
21. 0.036:1 or 3.6:100
22. 0.14%
23. 11.2%
24. 1.41:1
25. 1:0.18
26. 3.55%
27. 5.55
28. 1:0.28
29. $\frac{s}{a} = 0.002$ or $\frac{a}{s} = \frac{1}{0.002}$
30. 1:0.98

11 Dealing with Reconstitutions

Certain medications including penicillins and other antibiotics are unstable when stored in solution form and are therefore packaged in powder form. The dry powders must be reconstituted with a sterile diluent such as sterile water for injection (SWI) or sterile sodium chloride (normal saline; NS) solution. Instructions supplied with the vial indicate the volume of diluent to be added to adjust the desired strength. The resulting volume of the reconstituted drug and the approximate average concentration per milliliter are provided on the label or the package information sheet (known as *package insert*).

The powdered drug may or may not contribute to the final volume of the reconstituted solution in addition to the amount of diluent added. If the dry powder adds to the final volume of the reconstituted solution, the increase in volume obtained by the drug must be taken into account when calculating the amount of solvent to be used in preparing a solution of specified strength.

Some common problems regarding reconstitution of dry powders are provided in the following examples.

Example 1:

Assuming that the dry powder does not contribute to the final volume, how many milliliters of the reconstituted solution must be used to obtain the 3,000,000 IU of long-acting penicillin from original concentration of 12,000,000/5mL.

Solution:

No. of Units	*Volume (mL)*
1.2×10^7	5
3×10^6	x

by solving the proportion:

$$X\,(\text{mL}) = \frac{5 \times 3 \times 10^6}{1.2 \times 10^7} = 1.25\ mL$$

$\therefore 1.25\ mL$ *will contain* $3{,}000{,}000$ *IU of long-acting penicillin*

Example 2:

Assuming that the dry powder does not contribute to the final volume, how many milliliters of the reconstituted solution must be used to obtain the 600,000 IU of penicillin G sodium from original concentration of 1,000,000/5 mL.

Solution:

No. of Units	*Volume (mL)*
1×10^6	5
6×10^5	x

by cross multiplication:

$$X\,(\text{mL}) = \frac{5 \times 6 \times 10^5}{1 \times 10^6} = 3\ mL$$

$\therefore$ *3 mL will contain* 600,000 *IU of penicillin G sodium*

Example 3:

Using a vial of 500,000 units of penicillin G sodium and sodium chloride as diluent, explain how you would obtain the required units of penicillin G sodium to compound the following prescription:

℞

Penicillin G sodium	20,000 units/mL
Sodium chloride ad	10 mL
Sig. For iv injection	

Solution:

The total penicillin G sodium needed in the prescription

$$= 20{,}000 \times 10 = 200{,}000 \text{ units}$$

Since the dry powder represents 500,000 units of penicillin G sodium or 2.5 (500,000/200,000) times the amount required, 40% (200,000/500,000 × 100) of the powder will contain the prescribed number of units. Therefore, dissolve the dry powder of penicillin G sodium in a small quantity of sodium chloride and adjust the volume to 5 mL. Withdraw 2 mL from the reconstituted solution (which has the required number of penicillin units) and to this add 8 mL of saline to obtain 10 mL needed for injection.

PRACTICE PROBLEMS

1. Assuming that the dry powder does not contribute to the final volume, how many milliliters of the reconstituted solution must be used to obtain the 6,000,000 IU of long-acting penicillin from an original concentration of 12,000,000/5 mL?
2. Assuming that the dry powder does not contribute to the final volume, how many milliliters of the reconstituted solution must be used to obtain the 3,000,000 IU of long-acting penicillin from an original concentration of 12,000,000/4 mL?
3. A pharmacist receives a medication order for 600,000 units of penicillin G sodium to be added to one liter of D5W. A vial of penicillin G sodium containing a million units is on hand, and the directions on this vial state, "Add 5 milliliters of sterilized water for 2×10^5 units/mL". How many milliliters of the reconstituted solution must be added to the D5W to provide the desired concentration?
4. A pharmacist receives a medication order to prepare different concentrations of penicillin G potassium to be added to 1000 mL of D5W, using stock vials of 1,000,000 units of penicillin G sodium. The instructions on the vials of penicillin G potassium stated, "Add 4.6 milliliters of sterilized water for a concentration of 2.5×10^5 units/mL." How many milliliters of the reconstituted solution must be added to the D5W to provide the following units of penicillin G sodium in the final preparation?
   a. 2×10^5 units
   b. 4×10^5 units
   c. 5×10^5 units
   d. 6×10^5 units
   e. 2×10^6 units
   f. 1×10^6 units
5. Using a vial containing 300,000 units of penicillin G potassium, how many milliliters of sterile water for injection should be added to the dry powder in preparing a solution having a concentration of 30,000 units/mL?
6. Using a vial containing 300,000 units of penicillin G sodium, how many milliliters should be added to the dry powder in preparing a solution having a concentration of 25,000 units/mL?
7. Using a vial containing 12 million units of long-acting penicillin, how many milliliters of sterile water for injection should be added to the dry powder in preparing a solution having concentration of 2,000,000 units/mL?
8. Using a vial containing 1,000,000 units of penicillin G sodium, how many milliliters of diluent should be added to the dry powder in preparing a solution having a concentration of 250,000 units/mL?
9. Assuming that the dry powder does not contribute to the final volume, how many milliliters of the reconstituted solution must be used to obtain 300,000 IU of penicillin G potassium from original concentration of 1,000,000/2 mL?

***Note:* For the following questions, multiple answers are possible.**

10. Using a vial of 5,000,000 units of penicillin G sodium and normal saline as diluent, how would you obtain the required units of penicillin G sodium to compound the following prescription?

    ℞

Penicillin G sodium	40,000 units/mL
Normal saline ad	10 mL

    Sig. For IV injection.

11. Using a vial of 5,000,000 units of penicillin G potassium and normal saline as diluent, how would you obtain the required units of penicillin G sodium to compound the following prescription?

    ℞

Penicillin G potassium	10,000 units/mL
Normal saline ad	25 mL

    Sig. For topical use.

12. Using a vial of 6,000,000 units of long-acting penicillin and sodium chloride as diluent, how would you obtain the required units of penicillin G sodium to compound the following prescription?

    ℞

Long-acting penicillin	200,000 units/mL
Sodium chloride ad	25 mL

    Sig. For topical use.

13. Using a vial of 12,000,000 units of long-acting penicillin and sodium chloride as diluent, how would you obtain the required units of penicillin G sodium to compound the following prescription?

    ℞

Long-acting penicillin	400,000 units/mL
Sodium chloride ad	20 mL

    Sig. For topical use.

14. Using a vial containing 450,000 units of penicillin G potassium and sterile water for injection as a diluent, how would you prepare the following prescription?

    ℞

Long-acting penicillin	400,000 units/mL
Sodium chloride ad	20 mL

    Sig. For topical use.

15. Using a vial of 6,000,000 long-acting penicillin and water for injection as a diluent, how would you prepare the following prescription?

    ℞

Long-acting penicillin	60,000 units/mL
Water for injection ad	2 mL

    Sig. For IM injection

16. Using a vial containing 800,000 units of penicillin G potassium and sterile water for injection as a diluent, how would you prepare the following prescription?

    ℞

    Penicillin G potassium 40,000 units/mL
    Water for injection ad 5 mL
    Sig. For IM injection

17. A leaflet enclosed with a vial containing 6,000,000 units of penicillin G sodium states, "When 30 mL of sterile diluent are added the dry powder resulting concentration is 250,000 units/mL." Based on this information, how many milliliters of sterile water for injection should be used in preparing the following prescription?

    ℞

    Penicillin G potassium 6000,000 units
    Water for injection ad Q.S.
    Prepare a solution to contain 600,000 units/mL
    Sig. 1 mL = 600,000 units of penicillin G sodium

18. Neomycin sulfate is available in 1-g vials of maximum volume of 10 mL and the dry powder accounts for 0.9 mL of the final volume of the reconstituted product. Using a 1-g vial of neomycin sulfate and sterile water for injection as a diluent, how would you obtain the antibiotic concentration needed for the following prescription?

    ℞

    Neomycin sulfate 500 mg
    Water for injection ad 30 mL
    Sig. For topical use only.

19. The antibiotic streptomycin sulfate is in 5-g vial of 20 mL maximum capacity, for veterinary use, and the dry powder accounts for 5% increase of the final volume of reconstituted solution. Using a 5-g streptomycin sulfate vial and water for injection as a diluent, how would you obtain the antibiotic needed for the following prescription?

    ℞

    Streptomycin sulfate 1g
    Sodium chloride ad 100 mL
    Sig. For topical use only.

20. The information on the leaflets enclosed with a vial containing 5,000,000 units of penicillin G sodium states that when 23 mL saline diluent are added to the dry powder, the resulting concentration is 200,000 units/mL. Based on this information, how many milliliters of saline should be used in compounding 1,000,000 units of penicillin G sodium?

21. Using the contents of 5 mL vial of 1-g neomycin sulfate and sterile saline solution as a diluent, how would you obtain the neomycin sulfate required for the following prescription?

℞
Neomycin sulfate 400 mg
Sodium chloride ad 20 mL
Sig. Use as topical disinfectant.

22. A medication order calls for 600 mg of amoxicillin trihydrate to be administered IM to a pneumonic patient every 8 hours. Vials containing 250 mg, 500 mg, and 1 g of amoxicillin trihydrate are available. Based on the manufacturer's instructions, dilution may made as follows:

Drug Content/Vial	Volume of Diluent (mL)	Final Volume
¼ g	2	2.1
½ g	5	5.2
1 g	10	10.5

How could the prescribed dose of the antibiotic be obtained from each of the above three different potencies?

23. A medication order calls for 800 mg of Velosef to be administered IM to a pneumonic patient every 8 hours. Vials containing 250 mg, 500 mg, and 1 g of Velosef are available. On the basis of manufacturer's instructions, dilution may made as follows:

Drug Content/Vial	Volume of Diluent (mL)	Final Volume
¼ g	2	2
½ g	5	5
1 g	10	10

How could the prescribed dose of the antibiotic be obtained from the above three different potencies?

24. A medication order calls for 300 mg of Cephalexine to be administered IM to a pneumonic patient every 8 hours. Vials containing 500 mg, and 1 g of Cephalexine are available. Dilution may be made according to manufacturer's instructions as follows:

Drug Content/Vial	Volume of Diluent (mL)	Final Volume
½ g	5	5.2
1 g	10	10

How could the prescribed dose of the antibiotic be obtained from the above potencies?

25. Using the contents of a 5 mL vial of 1-g neomycin sulfate and sterile saline solution as a diluent, how would you obtain the neomycin sulfate required for the following prescription?

    ℞
    Neomycin sulfate 500 mg
    Sodium chloride ad 20 mL
    Sig. Use as topical disinfectant.

26. Using the contents of a 1,000,000-unit vial polymyxin B sulfate and sterile saline solution as a diluent, how would you obtain the antibiotic required to compound the following prescription?

    ℞
    Polymyxin B sulfate 200,000 units/mL
    Sodium chloride ad 30 mL
    Sig. Use as topical disinfectant.

27. A medication order calls for 1-g of amoxicillin monohydrate and sterile water for injection as a diluent, how would you obtain amoxicillin monohydrate needed to prepare the following prescription?

    ℞
    Amoxicillin monohydrate 500 mg
    Sodium chloride ad 15 mL
    Sig. Infantile suspension.
    15 drops to be taken orally every 8 hr.

28. Using a vial of 600 mg Velosef, how many milliliters of sterile water for injection should be added to the dry Velosef powder for preparing a solution having 150 mg/mL of the antibiotic Velosef?
29. Using a vial containing 750 mg of amoxicillin monohydrate, how many milliliters of water for injection should be added to the dry powder to prepare a solution having a concentration of 500 mg/mL of amoxicillin monohydrate? Assume that the dry powder does not contribute to the final volume.
30. For preparation of Augmentin (amoxicillin trihydrate and clavulanic acid as a potassium salt) oral suspension, 5 grams of the dry powder should be diluted with 45 mL of sterile water for injection to obtain a final solution containing 312 mg/mL. If the ratio between amoxicillin trihydrate and clavulanic acid as a potassium salt is 4:1, how much of each drug is present in 9 mL of suspension?
31. A medication order calls for 300 mg of Cefazolin sodium to be administered IM for a patient every 8 hours. Vials containing 250 mg and 500 mg are available. Based on the enclosed pamphlet's instructions, dilution can be made as follows:

Drug Content/Vial	Volume of Diluent (mL)	Final Volume
¼ g	2	2.1
½ g	2	2.2

How could the prescribed dose of the antibiotic be obtained from the above strengths?

32. A new hepatitis A vaccine offers a reduction in the number of doses to be taken. For this vaccine, vials containing 360 and 720 Enzyme-Linked Immunosorbent Assay (ELISA) units are available. According to the manufacturer's instructions, dilution may be made as follows:

No. of Units/Vial	Volume of Diluent (mL)	Final Volume
360	1	1.05
720	1	1.1

Based on the above information, how could a prescribed dose of 400 EL-U be obtained from the above strengths?

33. A new hepatitis A vaccine offers fewer doses to be taken. For this vaccine, vials containing 360 and 720 EL-U are available. According to the manufacturer's instructions, dilution may be made as follows:

No. of Units/Vial	Volume of Diluent (mL)	Final Volume
360	1	1.05
720	1	1.1

Based on the above information, how could a prescribed dose of 700 EL-U be obtained from the above strengths?

34. For a new hepatitis A vaccine that offers fewer doses to be taken, vials containing 1440 EL-U are available. According to the manufacturer's instructions, the dose will be ready after adding 2 mL of the diluent to the dry lyophilized powder. The final volume is expected to be 10% more upon reconstitution. Based on this information, how can the following doses be obtained?
    a. 1000 EL-U
    b. 1500 EL-U
    c. 850 EL-U
    d. 1250 EL-U

35. According to the package insert enclosed with a penicillin G potassium vial, the reconstituted solution is prepared by dissolving 250,000 units and the dry powder accounts for 1 mL increase in the final volume. Based on this information, how would you obtain the antibiotic required to compound the following prescription?

    ℞

Penicillin G potassium	250,000 units
Diluent ad	Q.S.

    Make solution containing 25,000 units/mL

36. A pharmacist has received a medication order for 100,000 units of penicillin G sodium to be added to 250 mL of D5W. A vial of penicillin G sodium containing one million units is on hand and the direction on the vial states, "Add 44.8 mL of sterile water for injection to obtain a concentration of 200,000 units/mL." How many milliliters of the reconstituted solution should be withdrawn and added to the D5W?

ANSWERS

1. 2.5 mL
2. 1 mL
3. 3 mL
4. a. 0.8 mL
   b. 1.6 mL
   c. 2 mL
   d. 2.4 mL
   e. 8 mL
   f. 4 mL
5. 10 mL
6. 12 mL
7. 6 mL
8. 4 mL
9. 0.6 mL

Note. For many of the following questions, multiple answers are possible.

10. Use 5 mL for reconstitution, then withdraw 4 mL and adjust the volume to 10 mL with normal saline.
11. Use 5 mL for reconstitution, then withdraw 2.5 mL with normal saline.
12. Use 6 mL for reconstitution, then withdraw 5 mL and adjust the volume to 25 mL with normal saline.
13. Use 6 mL for reconstitution, then withdraw 4 mL and adjust it to 20 mL with normal saline.
14. Use 3 mL for reconstitution, then withdraw 1 mL and adjust the volume to 5 mL with normal saline.
15. Use 50 mL for reconstitution, then withdraw 1 mL and adjust the volume to 2 mLwith normal saline.
16. Use 4 mL for reconstitution, then withdraw 1 mL and adjust the volume to 5 mL with normal saline.
17. 24 mL
18. Use 9.1 mL for reconstitution, then withdraw 5 mL and adjust the volume to 30 mL with normal saline.
19. Use 19 mL for reconstitution, then withdraw 4 mL and adjust the volume to 100 mL with normal saline.
20. 5 mL
21. Use 5 mL for reconstitution, then withdraw 2 mL and adjust the volume to 20 mL with normal saline.

22. 5.04 mL of ¼ g vial, 6.24 mL of ½ g vial, and 6.3 mL of 1g vial
23. 6.4 mL of ¼ g vial, 8 mL of ½ g vial, and 8 mL of 1g vial
24. 1.26 mL of ½ g vial, and 0.63 mL of 1g vial
25. Use 5 mL for reconstitution, then withdraw 2.5 mL and adjust the volume to 20 mL with normal saline.
26. Use 10 mL for reconstitution, then withdraw 5 mL and adjust the volume to 30 mL with normal saline.
27. Use 5 mL for reconstitution, then withdraw 2.5 mL and adjust the volume to 15 mL with normal saline.
28. 4 mL
29. 1.5 mL
30. 2246.4 mg of amoxicillin trihydrate and 561.6 mg of clavulanic acid as potassium salt
31. 2.52 mL of ¼ g vial and 1.32 mL of ½ g vial
32. 1.17 mL of 360 EL-U g vial and 0.611 mL of 720 EL-U vial
33. 2.04 mL of 360 EL-U g vial and 1.07 mL of 720 EL-U vial
34. a. 1.53 mL
    b. 2.3 mL
    c. 1.3 mL
    d. 1.91 mL
35. Use 9 mL for reconstitution to give a final volume of 10 mL containing 25,000 U of penicillin G potassium/mL
36. 0.5 mL

12 Determining Milliequivalent Strengths

The use of electrolyte solutions is very common in pharmacy practice. In hospital situations, various electrolyte solutions are administered to correct electrolyte imbalances. The concentrations of electrolyte solutions are generally expressed in chemical units known as *milliequivalents* (mEq), which represent the amount, in mg, of a solute equal to 1/1000 of its gram equivalent weight. A milliequivalent is a unit of measurement of the amount of chemical activity of an electrolyte. A milliequivalent unit is related to the total number of ionic charges in solution and it takes the valence of the ions into consideration.

Concentrations of electrolytes in body fluids and in pharmaceutical solutions are usually expressed as mEq/L or Eq/L. The normal electrolyte concentrations of cellular compartments are listed in Table 12.1, where values are expressed in mEq/L. Under normal conditions, plasma contains 155 mEq of cations and 155 mEq of anions. The total concentration of cations always equals the concentration of anions. Any number of mEq of Na^+, K^+, Ca^{2+}, Mg^{2+}, or any cation always reacts with precisely the same number of mEq of Cl^-, HCO_3^-, HPO_4^{2-}, SO_4^{2-}, or any other anion.

DOSAGE CALCULATIONS INVOLVING MILLIEQUIVALENTS

Clinically, the concentration of electrolytes in body fluids is expressed in mEq/L of fluid, and doses are calculated either in mEq or in metric weights. The relationship between mEq and the mg quantity of a substance can be expressed as follows:

$$\text{Weight of the substance in mg} = \text{Number of milliequivalents} \times \text{Milliequivalent weight}$$

In certain situations, the desired milliequivalents of electrolytes are obtained from stock solutions prepared at a known strength. In such cases, the following form of the expression can be used to calculate the number of milliequivalents:

$$\text{Number of mEq} = \frac{\text{Weight of the substance in mg}}{\text{Milliequivalent weight}}$$

If the milliequivalent concentration of a solute from a given solution needs to be determined, it can be obtained using the following expression:

$$\text{mE/L} = \frac{\text{Concentration of the solute in 1000 mL (g/L)}}{\text{Molecular weight (g/mol)}} \times \text{Valence} \times 1000$$

TABLE 12.1
Electolyte Composition of Cellular Compartments

	Extracellular Plasma	Interstitial	Intracellular
Na^+	143	146	15
K^+	5	5	150
Ca^{++}	5	3	2
Mg^{++}	2	1	27
Total cations	155	155	194
Cl^-	104	144	1
$HCO3^-$	27	30	10
$HPO4^=$	2	2	100
$SO4^=$	1	1	20
Organic acids	5	8	0
Proteinate	16	0	63
Total anions	155	155	194

Equivalent weights may be calculated for molecules as well as atoms using the expression:

$$\text{Equivalent weight} = \text{Atomic weight/Valence}$$

Valance, atomic, or formula weight and milliequivalent weights of most selected ions are summarized in Table 12.2. The equivalent weight of monovalent ions (such as sodium and chlorine) is identical to its molecular weight. The equivalent weight of NaCl is the sum of the equivalent weights of sodium (23 g/Eq) and chlorine (35.5 g/Eq), i.e., 58.5, which is identical to its molecular weight. However, the equivalent weight of a molecule having atoms that are not monovalent is different from its molecular weight. For example, the equivalent weight of Na_2CO_3 is 53 g/Eq, or half its molecular weight of 106. This circumstance can be explained as follows:

The molecule has two sodium atoms, each with an atomic weight of 23 ($23 \times 2 = 46$); these have a total valence of two and an equivalent weight of 23 g/Eq. The carbonate ion has a molecular weight of 60 and a valence of 2, and, therefore, an equivalent weight of 30 g/Eq. The equivalent weight of Na_2CO_3 molecule is sum of the equivalent weights of both ions in the molecule, i.e., 53 (23 + 30) g/Eq. The equivalent weight of a bivalent compound, thus, can be determined by dividing the sum of molecular or atomic weights of all atoms in the radical by the total valence of the positive or negative radical.

TABLE 12.2
Valence, Atomic, and Formula Weight and Milliequivalent Weights of Ions

Ion/Formula	Valence	Atomic Weight	mEq Weight
Lithium (Li^+)	1	7	7
Ammonium (NH_4^+)	1	18	18
Sodium (Na^+)	1	23	23
Chloride (Cl^-)	1	35.5	35.5
Potassium (K^-)	1	39	39
Acetate ($C_2H_3O_2^-$)	1	59	59
Bicarbonate (HCO_3^-)	1	61	61
Lactate ($C_3H_5O_3^-$)	1	89	89
Gluconate ($C_6H_{11}O_7^-$)	1	195	195
Phosphate ($H_2PO_4^-$)	1	97	97
Phosphate (HPO_4^{2-})	2	96	48
Magnesium (Mg^{2+})	2	24	12
Calcium (Ca^{2+})	2	40	20
Ferrous (Fe^{2+})	2	56	28
Carbonate (CO_3^{2-})	2	60	30
Sulfate (SO_4^{2-})	2	96	48
Aluminum (Al^{3+})	3	27	8
Ferric (Fe^{3+})	3	56	18.7
Citrate ($C_6H_5O_7^{2-}$)	3	189	63

Milliequivalent calculations of complex salts may be trickier sometimes. For a complex salt such as potassium acid phosphate (KH_2PO_4; molecular weight 136 g), the equivalent weight depends on how the compound is utilized. For potassium content, for example, the equivalent weight is identical to its molecular weight, i.e., 136 g. However, when used for its phosphate content, the equivalent weight is one third of the molecular weight. i.e., 136/3 = 45.3 g, since the valence of phosphate is 3. Similarly, when used for its hydrogen content in the preparation of buffers, the equivalent weight is one half the molecular weight, i.e., 136/2 = 68 g as it has two hydrogen atoms.

Note that when a quantity of binary compound (e.g., KCl or $CaCl_2.2H_2O$) is in a volume of solution, each radical will have exactly the same concentration when expressed in milliequivalents, but the solution will not contain the same weight of each radical. To compute the equivalent weight concentration of a salt hydrate in solution, the milligram weight of the water molecules must be included in the expressed milligram concentration of the salt.

Example 1:

How many milliequivalents of calcium ions are represented in a solution containing 40 mg calcium in 100 mL?

Solution:

For Ca^{2+}: $$\frac{0.400 \times 1000 \times 2 \times 1}{147} = 5.44 \; mEq \; of \; Ca^{++}$$

Example 2:

What is the milliequivalence of sodium chloride?

Solution:

$$Molecular\ weight\ of\ NaCl = 23 + 35.5 = 58.5$$

$$For\ NaCl,\ there\ is\ one\ pair\ of\ charge;$$

$$thus\ there\ is\ one\ equivalent/mol\ of\ NaCl.$$

$$Equivalent\ weight\ of\ NaCl = 58.5 \div 1 = 58.5\ \ g/mol$$

$$mEq\ of\ NaCl = 0.0585\ g$$

$$= 58.5\ mg$$

Example 3:

Sodium (Na^+) has an atomic weight of 23; what is the milliequivalence of sodium?

Solution:

First step:

Calculate the Eq. wt using this formula

$$Eq.wt = \frac{atomic\ weight}{valence}\ g/Eq.wt$$

$$\because For\ Na,\ the\ valence = 1$$

$$Eq.wt\ Na = \frac{23}{1} = 23\,g$$

Second step:

Calculate the mEq. wt using the formula:

$$mEq.\ wt = \frac{Eq.\ wt}{1000} = \frac{23}{1000}$$

$$= 0.023g = 23\,mg/mEq$$

Example 4:

A solution containing 526.5 mg of NaCl/dL has how many mEq of Na^+ and Cl^-?

Solution:

$$mEq.\ wt = 23 + 35.5 = 58.5\ mg/mEq$$

$$mEq = \frac{526.5\ mg}{58.5\ mg/mEq} = 9\ mEq\ of\ \text{NaCl}$$

which dissociates to 9 mEq of Na^+ and 9 mEq of Cl^-

PRACTICE PROBLEMS

1. A solution contains 521.5 mg of KCl in 100 mL. How many mEq of K^+ and Cl^- ions are present in this solution?
2. A prescription order calls for a 750 mL solution of potassium sulfate (K_2SO_4) containing 15 mEq of K^+. How many milligrams of potassium sulfate are needed?
3. A prescription order calls for a 500 mL solution of NaCl containing 10 mEq of Na^+. How many milligrams of NaCl are required?
4. How many mEq of Ca^{2+} are represented in a 500-mg tablet of calcium gluconate (molecular weight = 235 g/mol)?
5. How many mEq of K^+ are represented in a 500-mg tablet of potassium phenoxymethyl penicillin (molecular weight = 388 g/mol; valence = 1)?
6. What is the mEq wt of ferrous ion (Fe^{2+} ; g-atomic wt of 55.85 g)?
7. What is the mEq wt of sodium phosphate ($Na_2HPO_4.7H_2O$)?
8. How many mEq of Na^+ are in 120 mL of an 8% solution of sodium cyclamate (molecular weight = 201.33 g/mol; valence = 1)?
9. How many mEq of Ca^+ are available in a 500-mg tablet of calcium lactate pentahydrate (molecular weight = 308.3; valence = 2)?
10. How many mEq of Ca^+ are available in 400 mL of a solution of calcium chloride at 1.5 mg/mL strength?
11. How many milligrams of calcium chloride dihydrate ($CaCl_2 \cdot 2H_2O$, molecular weight = 147 g/mol) are needed to prepare 1500 mL of solution containing 5 mEq/liter Ca^{+2}?
12. How many milligrams of calcium chloride ($CaCl_2$, molecular weight = 111 g/mol) are needed to prepare 750 mL of solution containing 10 mEq/L of Ca^{+2}?
13. How many milligrams of sodium chloride are required to prepare 500 mL of solution containing 50 mEq/L of sodium?
14. How many mEq of potassium chloride are represented in 10-mL dose of 10% (w/v) potassium chloride syrup?
15. How many mEq of magnesium sulfate (molecular weight = 120) are represented in 30-mL dose of a 20% (w/v) magnesium sulfate extemporaneous laxative preparation?

16. How many mEq of potassium sulfate are represented by 15 mL of 25% potassium sulfate solution?
17. How many mEq of NaCl are represented by 3 g of NaCl?
18. How many mEq of potassium sulfate are represented by 870 mg of potassium sulfate?
19. A dehydrated patient has been receiving 1.5 mEq of sodium chloride per lb of his body weight. If this patient's body weigh is 150 lb, how many milliliters of 0.9% sterile saline solution should be given to this patient?
20. A patient has been receiving 3 mEq of sodium chloride per kg of his body weight. If this patient weighs 70 kg, how many milliliters of 0.9% sterile saline solution should be administered to this patient?
21. What is the Na^+ content in terms of mEq/L of a solution that contains 9 g of sodium chloride in a liter solution?
22. How many mEq of K^+ and Cl^- ions are available in 100 milliliters of a solution that contains 260.75 mg of KCl?
23. A prescription order calls for 750 mL solution of potassium sulfate to be made so that it will contain 7.5 mEq of K^+ ion. How many milligrams of potassium sulfate (K_2SO_4; molecular weight = 174 g/mol) are needed?
24. A prescription order calls for 500 mL solution of NaCl to be made so that it will contain 7.5 mEq of Na.$^+$ How many milligrams of NaCl are required?
25. How many mEq of Ca^{2+} are represented by 2 g of calcium chloride?
26. How many mEq of K^+ are in a 700-mg tablet of potassium phenoxymethyl penicillin (molecular weight = 388 g/mol; valence = 1)?
27. What is the mEq wt of sodium phosphate ($Na_2HPO_4 \cdot 7H_2O$)?
28. How many mEq of Na^+ are in 360 mL of an 8% solution of sodium cyclamate (molecular weight = 201.33 g/mol; valence = 1)?
29. How many mEq of Ca^+ are available in 750-mg calcium lactate pentahydrate (molecular weight = 308.3, valence = 2) tablet?
30. How many mEq of Ca^+ are available in 1200 mL of a solution of calcium chloride containing 1.5 mg/mL of Ca^+?
31. How many milligrams of calcium chloride dihydrate $CaCl_2 \cdot 2H_2O$ (molecular weight = 147 g/mol), are needed to prepare 500 mL of solution containing 5mEq/liter Ca^{+2}?
32. How many milligrams of calcium chloride ($CaCl_2$, molecular weight = 111 g/mol) are needed to prepare 750 mL of solution containing 5 mEq/L of Ca^{+2}?
33. How many mEq of potassium chloride are represented in a 10-mL dose of 20% (w/v) potassium chloride syrup?
34. How many mEq of magnesium sulfate (molecular weight = 120) are represented in each 30-mL dose of a 10% (w/v) magnesium sulfate extemporaneous laxative preparation?
35. How many mEq of potassium sulfate (K_2SO_4, molecular weight = 174) are available in 150 mL of 25% solution of potassium sulfate?
36. How many mEq of NaCl are available in 2.93-g of NaCl?

37. How many mEq of potassium sulfate (K_2SO_4, molecular weight = 174), are available in 3.480 g of potassium sulfate?
38. A dehydrated patient receives 1.5 mEq of sodium chloride per lb of his body weight. If the patient's body weighs 75 lb, how many milliliters of 0.9% sterile saline solution should the patient be given?
39. A patient receives 3-mEq of sodium chloride per kg of his body weight. If the patient weighs 140 kg, how many milliliters of 0.9% sterile saline solution should the patient be administered?
40. What is the Na^+ content in mEq/L of a solution containing 27 g of sodium chloride/liter solution?
41. A solution that contains 1.341 g of KCl has how many mEq of K^+ and Cl^-?
42. A prescription order calls for 1500 mL solution of potassium sulfate to be made so that it will contain 15 mEq of K^+ ion. How many milligrams of potassium sulfate (K_2SO_4, molecular weight = 174 g/mol) are needed?
43. A prescription order calls for one-liter solution of NaCl to be made so that it will contain 15 mEq of Na^+ ion. How many milligrams of NaCl (molecular weight = 58.5 g/mol) are required?
44. How many mEq of Na^+ are in 360 mL of 16% solution of sodium cyclamate (molecular weight = 201.33 g/mol, valence = 1)?
45. How many mEq of Ca^+ are available in 1200 mL of a solution of calcium chloride containing 3 mg/mL of Ca^+?
46. How many milligrams of calcium chloride ($CaCl_2$, molecular weight = 111 g/mol) are needed to prepare 3000 mL of solution containing 5 mEq/L of C^{+2}?
47. How many mEq of potassium chloride are represented in a 50-mL dose of 10% (w/v) potassium chloride syrup?
48. How many mEq of magnesium sulfate (molecular weight = 120) are represented in each 90-mL dose of a 15% (w/v) magnesium sulfate extemporaneous laxative preparation?

ANSWERS

1. 7 mEq each of potassium and chloride ions
2. 1305 mg
3. 585 mg
4. 4.26 mEq of Ca^{2+}/tablet
5. 1.29 mEq of K^+/tablet
6. 27.93 mg/mEq
7. 134 mg/mEq
8. 47.68 mEq/120 mL of 8% solution
9. 3.24 mEq Ca^{2+}/tablet
10. 10.81 mEq of Ca^+
11. 551.25 mg of $CaCl_2.2H_2O$
12. 416.25 mg
13. 1463 mg
14. 13.42 mEq
15. 100 mEq of $MgSO_4$
16. 43.1 mEq/15 mL of 25% solution of K_2SO_4
17. 51.3 mEq
18. 10 mEq
19. 1462.5 mL
20. 1365 mL
21. 153.9 mEq
22. 3.5 mEq
23. 652.5 mg

24. 438.75 mg
25. 36 mEq
26. 1.72 mEq of K^+/tablet
27. 134 mg/mEq
28. 143.04 mEq
29. 4.87 mEq Ca^{2+}/tablet
30. 32.43 mEq of Ca^+
31. 183.75 mg
32. 208.125 mg
33. 26.85 mEq
34. 50 mEq
35. 431 mEq
36. 50 mEq
37. 40 mEq
38. 731.25 mL
39. 2730 mL
40. 461.5 mEq
41. 18 mEq
42. 1305 mg
43. 877.5 mg
44. 286.1 mEq
45. 63.71 mEq
46. 832.5 mg
47. 67.1 mEq
48. 225 mEq

13 Dealing with Calories

Nutritional energy values are usually measured in kilocalories (kcal; or simply calories). One kilocalorie represents the amount of heat required to raise the temperature of 1 kilogram of water by 1°C at room temperature. In the metric system, the energy value is expressed in joules (J), with 1 kcal being equal to 4.184 kilojoules (KJ).

Glucose (dextrose) is the most commonly used energy substrate for TPN and may serve as the only nonprotein source of calories during TPN. The calories are also supplied by proteins and fats. The caloric density (kcal/g) of different nutritional substrates are listed in Table 13.1.

The calories represented by large volume parenterals and TPN products may be calculated in three steps as follows:

Step 1. Find the weight in g of each nutritional substrate in a specified volume of solution (or liquid preparation) using the following expression:

$$\text{g of nutritional substrate} = \text{Volume in mL} \times \text{Percent expressed as decimal}$$

Step 2. Find the calories represented by each nutritional substrate by multiplying the weight in g with its caloric density.

Step 3. Add the calories represented by all the nutritional substrates in the preparation.

Example 1:

How many calories are contained in 3 liters of D5W?

D5W is 5% dextrose in water
5% expressed as decimal = 0.05

Step 1. 3000 mL × 0.05 = 150 g
Step 2. 150 g × 3.4 kcal/g = 510 kcal, answer

Alternatively, the calories represented by large volume parenterals and TPN products may also be calculated by the method of proportion as follows:

D5W = dextrose 5% in water
If 100 mL contain 5 g, 3000 mL contain:

$$100 \text{ mL}/5 \text{ g} = 3000 \text{ mL}/X \text{ g}$$

$$X = 150 \text{ g}$$

$$150 \text{ g} \times 3.4 \text{ kcal} = 510 \text{ kcal, answer}$$

TABLE 13.1
Caloric Density of Nutritional Substrates

Nutritional Substrate	Caloric Density (kcal/g)
Glucose, anhydrous	3.85
Glucose, monohydrate	3.40
Proteins	4.10
Fat emulsions	9.0
Alcohol	7.0

Example 2:

How many calories are represented by a liter solution containing 20% dextrose, 12.5% proteins, and 5% fats?

Step 1. $1000 \times 0.2 = 200$ g dextrose
$1000 \times 0.125 = 125$ g proteins
$1000 \times 0.05 = 50$ g fats
Step 2. $200 \times 3.4 = 680$
$125 \times 4.1 = 512.5$
$50 \times 9 = 450$
Step 3. $680 + 512.5 + 450 = 1642.5$ kcal, answer

Example 3:

How many calories are represented by a liter solution containing 12.5% dextrose, 7.5% proteins, and 4.5% fats?

Step 1. $1000 \times 0.125 = 125$ g dextrose
$1000 \times 0.075 = 75$ g proteins
$1000 \times 0.045 = 45$ g fats
Step 2. $125 \times 3.4 = 425$
$75 \times 4.1 = 307.5$
$45 \times 9 = 405$
Step 3. $425 + 307.5 + 405 = 1137.5$ kcal, answer

PRACTICE PROBLEMS

1. How many calories are present in a 300-mL soft drink can that contains 1% fat?
2. How many calories would you obtain from 500 mL of a 2.5% glucose solution?
3. A parenteral mixture contains 5% dextrose and 2% sodium chloride. How many calories are provided by 2 liters of this mixture?
4. A patient in coma has been ordered 2000 kcal per day for survival. How many liters of a solution that contains 5% glucose and 5% fat are needed?
5. How many calories are present in a solution containing 25% NaCl solution?
6. If a person consumes 500 mL of 10% alcohol every day, what will be his weekly calorie intake from alcohol?
7. If a soup contains 30% vegetable protein, how many calories will be provided by 250 mL of this soup?
8. How many calories are represented by a 500 mL of 30% fat emulsion?
9. Mr. John Doe requires 2200 kcal per day for his anabolic needs. Assuming glucose as his only energy source, how much glucose does he need to take every day?
10. If a baked potato supplies 119 kcal, how many potatoes are needed to fulfill the daily energy requirement of 2261 kcal for a teenage girl?
11. If a normal healthy diet requires 0.8 g of protein per kg body weight per day, what will be the daily calorie gain of a 70-kg man from protein of a normal diet?
12. What is the total energy provided by a diet containing 50 g glucose, 20 g of protein, and 20 g of fat?
13. The daily energy requirement of a professional wrestler is 7000 kcal. If he is consuming carbohydrates equivalent to 1 kg of glucose, 500 g of meat protein and 100 g of fat everyday, how many more calories does he need to meet his requirement?
14. If 250 mL of an alcoholic beverage provides 175 calories, what is the strength of this solution in percent weight-by-volume (% w/v)?
15. How many calories are represented by one liter of a 25% glucose solution?
16. If the weight ratio of fat to water in an emulsion is 60:40 and if it provides 1080 kcal of energy, what is the total weight of this emulsion?
17. How many calories are in a chicken sandwich that contains starch equivalent to 20 g glucose, 10 g of protein, and 5 g of fat?
18. If a potato supplies 102 kcal from its glucose content, how much glucose does it contain?
19. How much protein is required if you would like to replace a diet of 500 g of glucose with protein?
20. In terms of caloric value, how much fat is equivalent to 900 g of glucose and 350 g of proteins?
21. How many calories are obtained from drinking 2 glasses of wine, if each glass contains 75 mL of 3.5% w/v of alcohol?

22. If an individual's daily consumption of protein is 50 g, how many calories does this individual gain solely from protein?
23. What would be your weekly energy consumption, if you eat 10 g of protein 3 times a day?
24. If the three members of a family consume 10, 20, and 30 g of fat each day, what would be their weekly total calorie intake from fat?
25. How much glucose is needed to get 1300 kcal of energy?
26. The daily calorie requirement for Ms. Thelma is 2600 kcal. If her daily intake is 300 g of glucose and 200 g of protein only, how much fat would she need to get the remaining energy?
27. How many calories are provided by a 250 mL solution containing 25% glucose and 10% sodium chloride?
28. If your daily energy requirement was met by 880 g of glucose, how much protein would you need to eat in order to meet the same energy requirement if you want to replace glucose with protein?
29. How much energy can three glasses of wine provide, if each contains 125 mL of 5% alcohol?
30. A mixture contains 200 g of glucose, 55 g of fat, and some protein. If the mixture provides 2000 kcal, how much protein is present in the mixture?

CALCULATIONS INVOLVING NITROGEN, CALORIE:NITROGEN RATIO, AND PROTEIN–CALORIE PERCENTAGE OF TPN PRODUCTS

Nitrogen

Nitrogen is an essential component of every tissue and organ system. For protein synthesis (anabolism) to occur, the diet must contain adequate nitrogen, usually in the form of protein. The adult requirement is approximately 0.8 to 1.5 g of protein/kg of body weight. Thus, a 70-kg adult may require between 56 to 105 g of protein every 24 hours in order to prevent negative nitrogen balance. One gram of nitrogen is contained in each 6.25 g of protein or amino acids (i.e., 16% of the total weight). A 70-kg adult will require between 9 and 17 g of nitrogen per 24 hours (i.e., 56/6.25 and 105/6.25).

Grams of nitrogen available from protein sources is calculated as follows:

$$\text{g of nitrogen} = \frac{\text{g of protein in solution}}{6.25}$$

Example 1:

Calculate g of nitrogen in 500 mL 8.5% amino acid solution.

8.5% = 8.5 g of amino acids/100 mL
500 mL would contain = 8.5 × 5 = 42.5 g of protein
g of nitrogen = 42.5/6.25 = 6.8 g, answer

Calorie:Nitrogen Ratio

The ratio of administered calories to grams of nitrogen should promote optimum nitrogen utilization for the synthesis of protein. The calorie:nitrogen (cal:N) ratio is determined by dividing the total non-nitrogen calories available with grams of nitrogen being provided. The optimal ratio is somewhere between 100 and 200 nonprotein calories per gram of nitrogen, with 135 to 175 being considered best for unstressed patients and slightly lower ratio for severely stressed patients.

Note. Do not take into account the calories from protein sources in computing calorie:nitrogen ratio.

Example 2:

Calculate calorie:nitrogen ratio of a TPN solution consisting of 500 mL of 50% dextrose and 500 mL of 8.5% amino acid solution.

$$\text{Nonprotein calories} = 50 \times 5 \times 3.4 = 850 \text{ kcal}$$

$$\text{g of amino acids (protein)} = 8.5 \times 5 = 42.5 \text{ g}$$

$$\text{g of nitrogen} = 42.5 \div 6.25 = 6.8 \text{ g}$$

$$\text{Ratio of non-nitrogen calories to g of nitrogen}$$

$$= 850 \text{ kcal} \div 6.8 \text{ g of N}$$

$$= 125{:}1, \text{ answer}$$

Protein–Calorie Percentage

The protein-calorie percentage of a TPN solution may be calculated as follows:

$$\text{Protein-calorie\%} = \frac{\text{Total \# of calories from protein sources}}{\text{Total \# of calories from all sources}} \times 100$$

Example 3:

Calculate protein-calorie percentage of a liter of 25% dextrose containing 4.25% amino acids.

$$250 \text{ g of dextrose} = 250 \times 3.4 \text{ kcal/g} = 850 \text{ kcal}$$

$$42.5 \text{ g of amino acids} = 42.5 \times 4 \text{ kcal/g} = 170 \text{ kcal}$$

$$\text{Total calories/liter} = 850 + 170 = 1020 \text{ kcal}$$

$$\text{Protein-calorie percentage of the solution}$$

$$= \frac{170}{1020} \times 100$$

$$= 16.7\%, \text{ answer}$$

PRACTICE PROBLEMS

1. How many calories are contained in 2.5 liters of 5% dextrose?
2. How many calories are represented by a liter of solution containing 15% dextrose, 10% proteins, and 8% fats?
3. A TPN solution consists of 0.75 liter of 10% dextrose and 0.25 liter of 4.25% amino acid solution. What is the ratio of non-nitrogen calories to grams of nitrogen for this TPN formula?
4. A TPN solution contains 0.5 liter of 25% dextrose and 0.5 liter of 8.5% amino acid solution. What is the ratio of non-nitrogen calories to grams of nitrogen for this TPN formula?
5. Calculate protein-calorie percentage of a liter of 10% dextrose containing 8.5% amino acids.
6. A liter TPN solution consists of 500 mL of 10% dextrose and 450 mL of 7.5% amino acids. What is the protein-calorie percentage of the solution?
7. A TPN solution consists of 500 mL of 25% dextrose and 500 mL of 10% amino acid solution.

   Calculate:
   a. The total number of calories present in the preparation.
   b. Grams of nitrogen in the preparation.
   c. The ratio of non-protein calories-to-grams of nitrogen.
   d. The protein-calorie percentage of the solution.

8. A patient is to receive one liter of the following admixture every 8 hours.

50% Dextrose in water	500 mL
8.5% Fre-Amine	500 mL

   Calculate:
   a. glucose calories/day
   b. grams of protein received/day
   c. grams of nitrogen received/day
   d. calorie-to-nitrogen ratio

9. Calculate the number of calories provided by a 250-mL solution containing 2% of fat, 25% of dextrose and 5.5% of protein.
10. How many milliliters of 20% dextrose solution or how many milliliters of 5% protein solution are required to get 50 kcal energy?
11. Calculate the amount of nitrogen present in 400 mL of 10% of an essential amino acid solution.
12. If a protein sample provides 2200 kcal of energy, how much nitrogen is present in it?
13. If a quantity of protein contains 50 g of nitrogen, how much energy can be generated from it?
14. How many milliliters of a 10% protein solution may contain 33 g of nitrogen?

15. If a person's daily energy requirement is 2000 kcal from protein sources, how much nitrogen should be present in his protein diet?
16. How much energy will be produced from a protein sample, which has 256 g of nitrogen?
17. How much nitrogen is present in a 250 mL solution containing 10% of protein X and 5% of protein Y.
18. If you eat a protein diet containing 30 g of nitrogen, how much energy will you get from it?
19. Calculate the number of grams of nitrogen present in a protein that provides 3300 kcal of energy.
20. How much nitrogen is present in 500 mL of a 33% protein solution?
21. Calculate the calorie:nitrogen ratio of a nutritional solution containing 500 g of glucose and 25 g of protein.
22. To maintain a calorie:nitrogen ratio of 150, how much protein should be taken with 220 g of fat diet?
23. If a diet contains 20 g of nitrogen, how much glucose would be needed to get a calorie:nitrogen ratio of 175?
24. If the energy gains of a person from protein diet and nonprotein diet are 180 and 900 kcal, respectively, what is the calorie:nitrogen ratio?
25. Calculate the calorie:nitrogen ratio of a diet containing 300 g of protein and 560 g of fat emulsion.
26. If the protein to nonprotein calorie ratio of a meal is 1:8, what is the calorie:nitrogen ratio?
27. A nutritional supplement contains 60% of dextrose, 5% fat, and 8% of protein. What will be its calorie:nitrogen ratio?
28. To keep a calorie:nitrogen ratio of 190, how much protein do you need to incorporate in a diet, which contains 200 g of fat?
29. If the calorie:nitrogen ratio of a meal is 180, how much dextrose should be taken with 25 g of protein?
30. What is the calorie:nitrogen ratio of a diet containing 99 g of fat and 81 g of protein?
31. What is the protein-calorie percentage of a solution containing 12% of dextrose and 5% of protein in 500 mL solution?
32. The protein-calorie percentage of a solution is 20%. If the total protein in it is 60 g, how many calories are supplied by the nonprotein fraction?
33. If the protein-calorie percentage of a meal is 25%, what is the ratio of calories from protein to nonprotein diet?
34. Calculate the protein-calorie percentage of a nutrition supplement containing 25 g of fat, 150 g of protein, and 80 g of dextrose.
35. What is the protein-calorie percentage of a 5-liter solution which contains 10% dextrose, 5% fat, and 15% protein?
36. Calculate the amount of nitrogen in a solution whose protein-calorie percentage is 33%. All nonprotein calories of this solution are solely provided by 35 g of fat.
37. How much protein should be incorporated in a diet containing 500 g of glucose to make a protein-calorie percentage of 15%?

38. Calculate the protein-calorie percentage of a 500 mL solution of 10% dextrose and 20% protein.
39. What is the protein-calorie percentage of a nutrition supplement containing 52 g of fat, 100 g of protein and 70 g of dextrose?
40. Calculate the amount of protein in a solution, whose protein-calorie percentage is 20% and which contains 400 g of dextrose.

ANSWERS

Calorie calculations

1. 27 kcal
2. 42.5 kcal
3. 340 kcal
4. 3.2 L
5. 0
6. 2450 kcal
7. 307.5 kcal
8. 1350 kcal
9. 647 g
10. 19
11. 229.6 kcal
12. 432 kcal
13. 650 kcal
14. 10%
15. 850 kcal
16. 200 g
17. 154 kcal
18. 30 g
19. 414.6 g
20. 499 g
21. 36.75 kcal
22. 205 kcal
23. 861 kcal
24. 3780 kcal
25. 382.4 g
26. 84.4 g
27. 212.5 kcal
28. 730 g
29. 131 kcal
30. 201 g

Nitrogen calculations, Calorie:Nitrogen ratio, and Protein–Calorie percentage

1. 425 kcal
2. 1640 kcal
3. 150
4. 62.5
5. 50.6%
6. 45%
7. See below
   a. 630 kcal
   b. 8 g
   c. 53
   d. 32.5%
8. See below
   a. 2550 kcal
   b. 127.5 g
   c. 20.4 g
   d. 125
9. 314 kcal
10. 73.5 mL, 244 mL
11. 6.4 g
12. 85.9 g
13. 1281 kcal
14. 2062.5 mL
15. 78 g
16. 6560 kcal
17. 6 g
18. 769 kcal
19. 129 g
20. 26.4 g
21. 425
22. 82.5 g
23. 1029 g
24. 128

25. 105
26. 205
27. 194.5
28. 59.2 g
29. 212 g
30. 69
31. 33.4%
32. 984 kcal
33. 1:3
34. 55.3%
35. 44%
36. 6 g
37. 73 g
38. 71%
39. 37%
40. 83 g

14 Determining Intravenous Flow Rates

Intravenous (IV) flow rate calculations are usually required in a hospital situation. By means of these calculations, the rate of flow of an IV medication can be determined to administer certain volume of liquid when the duration of administration is known. To calculate the rate of flow (rate of infusion) of IV solutions, one can use either the method of proportion (which generally involves two steps) or the formula method. In the formula method, the rate of infusion can be calculated as follows:

$$\text{Number of drops per minute (or gtt/min)} = \frac{\text{Volume of solution to be infused (mL)} \times \text{number of drops per mL (or drop factor)}}{\text{Number of hours for admin} \times 60 \text{ (minutes per hour)}}$$

The above formula can be simplified as:

$$R = \frac{V \times D}{T}$$

where

R = rate of flow (gtt/min)
V = total volume to be infused (in mL)
D = drop factor (gtt/mL)
T = total time of infusion (in minutes)

Note: A drop factor set of 60 drops per mL is referred to as a "microdrip" or "microdrop" set. When the drops are fewer than 60, e.g., 10 drops or 20 drops per mL, the set is referred to as "macrodrip" set. It is not very practical or common to have more than 60 drops per mL. However, sometimes, some higher drop factors are used only for calculations exercise.

Example 1:

One liter of an intravenous fluid was started in a patient at 6:00 A.M. and scheduled to run for 12 hours. At 1:00 P.M. it was found that 600 mL of the fluid remained in the bottle. At what rate of flow should the remaining fluid be regulated using an IV set that delivers 15 drops per mL in order to complete the administration of the fluid in the scheduled time?

Fluid remaining = 600 mL
Time remaining = 5 hr or 300 min

A. By formula method:

$$\text{Number of drops per minute (or gtt/min)} = \frac{600 \times 15}{5 \times 60}$$

$$= 30 \text{ drops/min}$$

B. By method of proportion:

Step 1. If 600 mL is infused in 300 minutes, how many milliliters will be infused in 1 minute?

$$\frac{600 \text{ mL}}{300 \text{ min}} = \frac{\text{X ml}}{1 \text{ min}}$$

$$\text{X} = 2 \text{ mL}$$

Step 2. If 15 drops were contained in 1 mL, how many drops would be contained in 2 mL?

$$\frac{15 \text{ drops}}{1 \text{ mL}} = \frac{\text{X drops}}{2 \text{ mL}}$$

$$\text{X} = 30 \text{ drops}$$

Answer: rate of flow = 30 drops per minute

Example 2:

The physician's order reads "500 cc D5W IV in 12 hours." How many drops per minutes should the IV infusion run if a microdrop administration set is used? The microdrop set delivers 60 gtt/mL.

A. By formula method:

$$\text{Number of drops per minute (or gtt/min)} = \frac{500 \times 60}{12 \times 60}$$

$$\text{X} = 41.67 \text{ or } 42 \text{ gtt/min}$$

B. By the method of proportion:

Step 1. If 500 mL is infused in 720 minutes, how many mL will be infused in 1 minute?

$$\frac{500 \text{ mL}}{720 \text{ min}} = \frac{\text{X mL}}{1 \text{ min}}$$

$$\text{X} = 0.69 \text{ mL}$$

Step 2. If 60 drops are contained in 1 mL, how many drops would be contained in 0.69 mL?

$$\frac{60 \text{ drops}}{1 \text{ mL}} = \frac{X \text{ drops}}{0.69 \text{ mL}}$$

$$X = 41.4 \text{ drops}$$

Answer: rate of flow = 41 drops per minute

Example 3:

If a physician prescribes 10 units of insulin to be added to a liter IV solution of D5W and administered to a patient over an 8-hr period, how many drops per min should be administered using an IV set that delivers 20 drops per mL?

A. By formula method:

$$\text{Number of drops per minute (or gtt/min)} = \frac{1000 \times 20}{8 \times 60}$$

$$X = 41.67 \text{ or } 42 \text{ drops/min}$$

B. By the method of proportion:

Step 1. If 1000 mL is infused in 1440 minutes, how many mL will be infused in 1 minute?

$$\frac{1000 \text{ mL}}{480 \text{ min}} = \frac{X \text{ mL}}{1 \text{ min}}$$

$$X = 2.08 \text{ mL}$$

Step 2. If 20 drops are contained in 1 mL, how many drops would be contained in 2.08 mL?

$$\frac{20 \text{ drops}}{1 \text{ mL}} = \frac{X \text{ drops}}{2.08 \text{ mL}}$$

$$X = 21 \text{ drops}$$

Answer: rate of flow = 41.6 or 42 drops per minute

PRACTICE PROBLEMS

1. Calculate the IV flow rate for 800 mL D5W to run for 4.5 hours. The drop factor is 60 gtt/mL. Solve the problem by formula and proportion methods.
2. Calculate the IV flow rate for 950 cc of 0.9% NaCl IV over 11.5 hours. The drop factor is 28 gtt/mL. Solve the problem by formula and proportion methods.
3. Calculate the IV flow rate for 900 mL D5W to run for 9 hours. The drop factor is 50 gtt/mL. Solve the problem by formula and proportion methods.
4. Calculate the IV flow rate for 800 cc of 0.9% NaCl IV over 9 hours. The drop factor is 50 gtt/mL. Solve the problem by formula and proportion methods.
5. Calculate the IV flow rate for 1000 mL D5W to run for 12 hours. The drop factor is 60 gtt/mL. Solve the problem by formula and proportion methods.
6. Calculate the IV flow rate for 1800 cc of 0.9% NaCl IV over 9 hours. The drop factor is 30 gtt/mL. Solve the problem by formula and proportion methods.
7. Calculate the IV flow rate for 9000 mL D5W to run for 12 hours. The drop factor is 60 gtt/mL. Solve the problem by formula and proportion methods.
8. Calculate the IV flow rate for 1600 cc of 0.9% NaCl IV over 12 hours. The drop factor is 40 gtt/mL. Solve the problem by formula and proportion methods.
9. Calculate the IV flow rate for 1600 mL D5W to run for 6 hours. The drop factor is 60 gtt/mL. Solve the problem by formula and proportion methods.
10. Calculate the IV flow rate for 4500 cc of 0.9% NaCl IV over 16 hours. The drop factor is 20 gtt/mL. Solve the problem by formula and proportion methods.
11. Calculate the IV flow rate for 500 mL D5W to run for 8 hours. The drop factor is 60 gtt/mL. Solve the problem by formula and proportion methods.
12. Calculate the IV flow rate for 200 cc of 0.9% NaCl IV over 2 hours. The drop factor is 20 gtt/mL. Solve the problem by formula and proportion methods.
13. Calculate the IV flow rate for 1500 mL D5W to run for 24 hours. The drop factor is 60 gtt/mL. Solve the problem by formula and proportion methods.
14. Calculate the IV flow rate for 1200 cc of 0.9% NaCl IV over 22 hours. The drop factor is 20 gtt/mL. Solve the problem by formula and proportion methods.
15. Calculate the IV flow rate for 2000 mL D5W to run for 8 hours. The drop factor is 60 gtt/mL. Solve the problem by formula and proportion methods.
16. Calculate the IV flow rate for 5000 cc of 0.9% NaCl IV over 24 hours. The drop factor is 20 gtt/mL. Solve the problem by formula and proportion methods.

17. Calculate the IV flow rate for 900 mL D5W to run for 6 hours. The drop factor is 60 gtt/mL. Solve the problem by formula and proportion methods.
18. Calculate the IV flow rate for 1300 cc of 0.9% NaCl IV over 24 hours. The drop factor is 20 gtt/mL. Solve the problem by formula and proportion methods.
19. Calculate the IV flow rate for 400 mL D5W to run for 6 hours. The drop factor is 60 gtt/mL. Solve the problem by formula and proportion methods.
20. Calculate the IV flow rate for 800 cc of 0.9% NaCl IV over 9 hours. The drop factor is 20 gtt/mL. Solve the problem by formula and proportion methods.
21. Calculate the IV flow rate of a liter of normal saline to be infused in 6 hours. The infusion set is calibrated for a drop factor of 15 gtt/mL. Solve the problem by formula and proportion methods.
22. A physician's order calls for 2000 mL D5W IV to run for 24 hours. If the infusion set is calibrated to 15 drops per milliliter, calculate the IV flow rate in gtt/min. Solve the problem by formula and proportion methods.
23. Calculate the IV flow rate of a liter of normal saline to be infused in 6 hours. The infusion set is calibrated for a drop factor of 30 gtt/mL. Solve the problem by formula and proportion methods.
24. Calculate the IV flow rate for 2 liter of normal saline to be infused in 12 hours. The infusion set is calibrated for a drop factor of 30 gtt/mL. Solve the problem by formula and proportion methods.
25. Calculate the IV flow rate of 6000 ml normal saline to be infused in 6 hours. The infusion set is calibrated for a drop factor of 45 gtt/mL. Solve the problem by formula and proportion methods.
26. Calculate the IV flow rate of 3000 mL normal saline to be infused in 24 hours. The infusion set is calibrated for a drop factor of 60 gtt/mL. Solve the problem by formula and proportion methods.
27. Calculate the IV flow rate of 4000 mL normal saline to be infused in 5 hours. The infusion set is calibrated for a drop factor of 50 gtt/mL. Solve the problem by formula and proportion methods.
28. Calculate the IV flow rate of 2500 mL normal saline to be infused in 10 hours. The infusion set is calibrated for a drop factor of 45 gtt/mL. Solve the problem by formula and proportion methods.
29. Calculate the IV flow rate of 5000 mL normal saline to be infused in 8 hours. The infusion set is calibrated for a drop factor of 55 gtt/mL. Solve the problem by formula and proportion methods.
30. Calculate the IV flow rate of a liter of normal saline to be infused in 48 hours. The infusion set is calibrated for a drop factor of 50 gtt/mL. Solve the problem by formula and proportion methods.
31. Calculate the IV flow rate of 600 mL normal saline to be infused in 24 hours. The infusion set is calibrated for a drop factor of 6 gtt/mL. Solve the problem by formula and proportion methods.
32. Calculate the IV flow rate of one-half liter normal saline to be infused in 2 hours. The infusion set is calibrated for a drop factor of 12 gtt/mL. Solve the problem by formula and proportion methods.

33. Calculate the IV flow rate of 3500 mL normal saline to be infused in 32 hours. The infusion set is calibrated for a drop factor of 45 gtt/mL. Solve the problem by formula and proportion methods.
34. Calculate the IV flow rate of 4000 mL of normal saline to be infused in 22 hours. The infusion set is calibrated for a drop factor of 20 gtt/mL. Solve the problem by formula and proportion methods.
35. Calculate the IV flow rate of a liter of normal saline to be infused in 2 hours. The infusion set is calibrated for a drop factor of 5 gtt/mL. Solve the problem by formula and proportion methods.
36. Calculate the IV flow rate of 5500 normal saline to be infused in 16 hours. The infusion set is calibrated for a drop factor of 15 gtt/mL. Solve the problem by formula and proportion methods.
37. Calculate the IV flow rate of 3500 mL normal saline to be infused in 32 hours. The infusion set is calibrated for a drop factor of 45 gtt/mL. Solve the problem by formula and proportion methods.
38. Calculate the IV flow rate of 4000 mL of normal saline to be infused in 22 hours. The infusion set is calibrated for a drop factor of 20 gtt/mL. Solve the problem by formula and proportion methods.
39. Calculate the IV flow rate of 3 liter of normal saline to be infused in 20 hours. The infusion set is calibrated for a drop factor of 50 gtt/mL. Solve the problem by formula and proportion methods.
40. Calculate the IV flow rate of 6500 normal saline to be infused in 12 hours. The infusion set is calibrated for a drop factor of 15 gtt/mL. Solve the problem by formula and proportion methods.

ANSWERS

1. 177 drops per minute
2. 39 drops per minute
3. 83 drops per minute
4. 74 drops per minute
5. 83 drops per minute
6. 100 drops per minute
7. 750 drops per minute
8. 89 drops per minute
9. 267 drops per minute
10. 94 drops per minute
11. 62.5 or 63 drops per minute
12. 33.3 or 33 drops per minute
13. 62.5 or 63 drops per minute
14. 18 drops per minute
15. 250 drops per minute
16. 69 drops per minute
17. 150 drops per minute
18. 18 drops per minute
19. 66.7 or 67 drops per minute
20. 30 drops per minute
21. 42 drops per minute
22. 20.8 drops per minute
23. 83 drops per minute
24. 83 drops per minute
25. 750 drops per minute
26. 125 drops per minute
27. 667 drops per minute
28. 188 drops per minute
29. 573 drops per minute
30. 17.4 or 17 drops per minute
31. 2.5 or 3 drops per minute
32. 50 drops per minute
33. 82 drops per minute
34. 60.6 or 61 drops per minute

35. 42 drops per minute
36. 86 drops per minute
37. 82 drops per minute
38. 60.6 or 61 drops per minute
39. 125 drops per minute
40. 135 drops per minute

15 Working with Insulin and Heparin Products

INSULIN

Insulin injections are very commonly prescribed for patients suffering from diabetes. It is expressed in *units of activity* per milliliter. For example, "insulin 10 units" means 10 units of insulin are present in 1 mL of the injection. Insulin should always be measured in insulin syringes, which are calibrated according to the strength of insulin. The insulin syringe makes it possible to obtain a correct dosage without any mathematical computations or conversions. Always use the smallest capacity insulin syringe possible to most accurately measure insulin dosages. The insulin dosages are calculated by the method of proportion. This is explained in the following examples.

WORKING WITH INSULIN STRENGTH

Insulin strength calculations are performed by ratios and proportions. Following are some common problems associated with insulin calculations.

Example 1:

A physician has prescribed 30 units of U-100 mixtard insulin and 45 Units of U-40 PZI (ilentin 1) insulin for a diabetic patient. What volumes in milliliters of each type of insulin should be administered to provide the prescribed dosage?

Solution:

A. For U-100 mixtard insulin:
Each mL contains 100 U.

No. of Units	Volume (mL)
100	1
30	x

$$X\ (\text{mL}) = \frac{1 \times 30}{100} = 0.30\ mL\ of\ U-100\ mixtard\ insulin$$

B. For U-40 PZI insulin:
Each mL contains 40 U.

No. of Units	Volume (mL)
40	1
45	x

$$X\ (\text{mL}) = \frac{1 \times 45}{40} = 1.1\ \textit{mL of } U-40 \textit{ isophane insulin}$$

Example 2:

How many units of U-100 protamine zinc insulin are available in 1.4 mL?

Solution:

No. of Units	Volume (mL)
100	1
X	1.4

$$X\ (\text{mL}) = \frac{1.4 \times 100}{1} = 140\ \textit{units of protamine zinc insulin}$$

Example 3:

A physician prescribed 3 units of subcutaneous insulin injection for every 25 mg% increase in the blood glucose level above 180 mg% twice a day. The patient's blood glucose level reads 255 and 310 mg% at the predetermined time intervals. How many total units of insulin should be injected to maintain the patient's normal blood glucose level?

Solution:

For 180 mg%:

$$255 - 180 = 75\ \text{mg\%}$$

$$3\ \text{units} = 25\ \text{mg\%}$$

$$X\ \text{units} = 75\ \text{mg\%}$$

$$X = 9\ \text{units}$$

For 310 mg%:

$$310 - 180 = 130 \text{ mg\%}$$

$$3 \text{ units} = 25 \text{ mg\%}$$

$$X \text{ units} = 130 \text{ mg\%}$$

$$X = 390/25 = 15.6 \text{ units}$$

PRACTICE PROBLEMS

Questions 1-16 have multiple choices. Select the best answer.

1. 1.5 mL of U-40 semilent contain:
   a. 45 units
   b. 60 units
   c. 55 units
   d. 80 units
2. 0.04 mL of concentrated U-500 Iletin® II contain:
   a. 20 units
   b. 200 units
   c. 100 units
   d. 40 units
3. 1.8 mL of isophane insulin contain:
   a. 70 units
   b. 82 units
   c. 80 units
   d. 72 units
4. 12 mL U-40 Lent Iletin I insulin contain:
   a. 1200 units
   b. 600 units
   c. 480 units
   d. 48 units
5. 7.5 mL U-100 NPH Iletin I contain:
   a. 7500 units
   b. 750 units
   c. 75 units
   d. 7.5 units
6. 0.32 mL of U-100 Humulin® N insulin contain:
   a. 320 units
   b. 32 units
   c. 300 units
   d. 30 units

7. How many milliliters of U-100 protamine zinc contain 500 units?
   a. 10 mL
   b. 15 mL
   c. 5 mL
   d. 7.5 mL
8. How many milliliters are needed to provide a dose of 400 units of U-40 regular Iletin I?
   a. 100 mL
   b. 10 mL
   c. 15 mL
   d. 200 mL
9. How many milliliters of U-40 Lent Iletin I are needed to give 600 units?
   a. 150 mL
   b. 15 mL
   c. 1.5 mL
   d. 30 mL
10. What volume of U-100 Humulin N insulin is required to provide 850 units?
    a. 8.5 μL
    b. 85 mL
    c. 85 μL
    d. 8500 μL
11. What is the volume of U-40 Lent Iletin insulin required to provide a 500-unit dose?
    a. 1250 μL
    b. 125 μL
    c. 125 mL
    d. 12500 μL
12. What volume of U-100 Novolin® insulin is needed to provide 1500 units?
    a. 150 mL
    b. 1500 mL
    c. 15000 mL
    d. 15000 μL
13. What volume of U-40 isophane insulin is required to provide 30 units?
    a. ½ mL
    b. ⅓ mL
    c. ¾ mL
    d. ⅔ mL
14. What volume of purified U-100 Insulatard® NPH insulin will provide 1600 units?
    a. 160 mL
    b. 160 μL
    c. 1600 mL
    d. 16000 μL
15. What volume of purified U-100 NPH insulin will be needed to provide a prescribed dose of 70 units?

a. 0.7 μL
b. 70 μL
c. 700 μL
d. 7000 μL

16. What volume of U-40 NPH Iletin I insulin will provide a prescribed dose of 90 units?
    a. 225 μL
    b. 2.25 mL
    c. 22.5 μL
    d. 0.225 mL
17. Calculate the total insulin dose in milliliters if the prescribed dose reads 0.02 mL/kg per day and the patient weighs 189 lb.
18. What is the total insulin daily dose in units if the prescribed dose reads 1.5 units/kg for a patient weighing 160 lb?
19. What is the total insulin daily dose in units if the prescribed dose reads 0.42 units/lb for a patient who weighs 72 kg?
20. What is the total insulin daily dose in milliliters if the prescribed dose reads 0.009 mL/kg and the patient weighs 245 lb?
21. What is the total insulin dose in milliliters if the prescribed dose reads one unit/lb per day and the patient weighs 95 kg?
22. What is the total insulin dose in milliliters if the prescribed dose reads 0.85 mL/10 kg per day and the patient weighs 210 lb?
23. A medication order in the hospital calls for U-500 concentrated Iletin I insulin to be administered to a 120-lb female patient on the basis of 0.1 units per pound/day. How many units of this product should be given to her daily?
24. A medication order in the hospital calls for U-500 concentrated Iletin I insulin to be administered to a 240-lb female patient on the basis of 0.2 units per pound/day. How many units of this product should be given to her daily?
25. A medication order in the Chenal Clinic calls for U-100 mixtard to be administered to a 300-lb patient on the basis of 10 mL/lb per day. How many mL of U-100 mixtard insulin should be given for this patient?
26. A medication order in the hospital calls for U-100 protamine zinc insulin to be administered to a 120-lb female patient on the basis of 0.5 units per pound/day. How many units of protamine zinc should be given to her daily?
27. A medication order in the clinic calls for U-100 mixtard to be administered to a 150-lb patient on the basis of 10 mL/lb per day. How many mL of U-100 mixtard insulin should be given for this patient?
28. A patient was receiving 2.5 mL/day of U-100 Humulin insulin. However, because of some hepatic and renal disorders, the dose was reduced by 70%. How many units of Humulin insulin will the patient receive now?
29. A medication order in a clinic for a 220-lb diabetic patient calls for humulin to be given on the basis of 2 units/kg. How many units of Humulin should be given?

30. A medication order in UAMS hospital calls for protamine zinc insulin to be administered to a 65-kg patient on the basis of 0.5 units/lb per day. How many units of protamine zinc should be administered daily?
31. A medication order in a hospital setting calls for U-100 velosulin insulin to be given to a patient of 150 lb on the basis of 1.5 units/kg per 24 hours. How many units of U-100 velosulin insulin should be administered daily?
32. What volume of protamine zinc should the patient receive a day, if his weight is 185 lb and the prescribed dose for him is 0.06/kg?
33. Dr. Doe has prescribed Mr. Foreman 0.4 mL U-100 mixtard (70% NPH:30% regular premix) insulin and 0.5 mL of U-40 isophane insulin. How many units of each type of insulin should the patient be receiving?
34. A patient is required to take 50 units of U-40 isophane insulin and 0.5 mL of U-100 protamine zinc. How many milliliters and units of each type are needed to provide the sufficient doses of the prescribed insulins?
35. A diabetic patient is required to take 1.5 mL of U-40 Lent insulin, and 0.7 mL of U-100 velosulin human insulin. How many units of each type of insulin would be contained in volumes taken?
36. A physician has prescribed 15 units of U-100 protamine zinc insulin suspension and 24 units of U-40 isophane insulin for a diabetic patient. What volumes, in milliliters, of each type will provide the prescribed dosages?
37. An insulin-dependent chronic diabetic patient is required to receive 25 units of U-40 regular Iletin I and 5 units of U-500 concentrated Iletin II. What volumes, in milliliters, of each type will be needed to provide the sufficient dosages?
38. To keep his blood glucose level normal, a diabetic patient is required to take 30 units of U-40 NPH Iletin and 80 units of U-100 Insulatard NPH. What volumes, in milliliters, of each kind of insulin are necessary to maintain the patient's normal blood glucose level?
39. How many units of U-40 isophane insulin are there in 0.75 mL?
40. A diabetic patient is required to receive 20 U of U-100 Humulin (human insulin) and 10 U of U-100 protamine zinc insulin. What volume, in milliliters, of each type of insulin should be administered to provide the prescribed dosage?
41. A hospital pharmacist is placing a monthly order for different types of insulins that have to be sufficient for 100 hospitalized patients. If each patient receives 10 mL/month of U-100 Humulin insulin and 15 mL/month of U-400 mixtard, how many units of each type should the pharmacist order to provide the amount needed for the 100 patients for the entire month?
42. How many units of U-100 Humulin are there in 2 mL?
43. A physician orders 0.125 mL of insulin injection subcutaneously for every 10 mg/mL of blood glucose above 180 mg/mL with blood glucose levels and injections taken three times/day (every 8 hr). The patient's blood glucose levels were 280 mg/mL, 260 mg/mL, and 320 mg/mL at the predetermined time intervals. What total volume of insulin injection

should be administered to maintain the patient's blood glucose level around normal level?

44. For a diabetic patient, the physician orders subcutaneous injection of U-40 isophane insulin, and 0.7 mL of U-100 mixtard insulin for every 100 mg/mL increase over 190 mg/mL with blood glucose level taken twice a day. If the patient's blood glucose level reads 480 mg/mL at morning and 340 mg/mL at evening, how many total units of both types of insulin should be given at the morning and at the evening to keep the patient's blood glucose at 190 mg/mL?
45. According to the physician's prescription, a diabetic patient was receiving 0.3mL of U-100 ultralent insulin and 0.2 mL of U-100 humulin insulin. How many units of each type of insulin should the patient be administered to provide the prescribed dosage?
46. A physician ordered 0.4 mL of subcutaneous for every 30 mg% of blood glucose injection over 170%, twice a day in the morning and evening. The patient's blood glucose levels were 300 and 350 mg% in the morning and evening, respectively. What total volume of insulin should be injected to keep the patient's normal blood glucose level?
47. In order to reduce the required insulin dose, a physician advised a chronic diabetic patient to follow a dietary regime and ordered 0.8 mL of U-40 NPH Iletin I and 0.5 mL of U-100 Humulin insulin. These doses are ¾ of the original doses before following the special food regime. How many units of each kind of insulin did the patient receive originally?
48. A chronic diabetic patient receives 70% of his insulin medication as U-40 isophane insulin and the remaining percentage as U-100 mixtard. If the total volume of the medication received by the patient is 2 mL, how many units of each type of insulin is the patient taking to maintain his normal blood glucose level?
49. A hospital pharmacist is planning to place an order for two different types of insulins including 1×10^6 units of U-100 Insulatard insulin and 4×105 units of U-40 NPH Iletin I insulin. How many vials of each type should the pharmacist order if the vial size available is 10 mL?
50. A hospital pharmacist was placed an order for 1.6×10^5 units of Isophane insulin. How many vials of this product should the pharmacist order if the vial size available is 10 mL?

HEPARIN DOSAGE

Similar to insulin, heparin is also measured in *units of activity*. However, heparin is used for blood thinning to prevent clot formation. Intravenous heparin may be administered by standard gravity flow or electronic infusion devices. The normal adult heparinizing dosage is 20,000–40,000 units per 24 hours. In general, IV heparin is ordered in units per hour or flow rate in milliliter per hour. The heparin dosages may be calculated by the method of proportion. This is explained in the examples that follow.

Example 1:

A heparin dose of 90 units/kg of body weight has been recommended for a patient undergoing certain type of surgery. How many mL of an injection containing 5000 heparin units/mL should be administered to a 180-lb patient?

$$90 \text{ units}/2.2 \text{ lb} = \text{X units}/180 \text{ lb}$$

$$\text{X} = 7364 \text{ units}$$

$$5000 \text{ units}/1 \text{ mL} = 7364 \text{ units}/\text{X}$$

$$\text{X} = 1.47 \text{ mL, answer}$$

Example 2:

A patient is to receive an IV drip of the following:

Sodium Heparin	10,000 units
Normal saline	500 mL

a. How many milliliters per hour must be administered to achieve a rate of 1200 units of sodium heparin per hour?

$$10{,}000 \text{ units}/500 \text{ mL} = 1200 \text{ units}/\text{X}$$

$$\text{X} = 60 \text{ mL per hour, answer}$$

b. If the IV set delivers 15 drops/mL, how many drops per minute should be administered?

Number of drops per minute (or gtt/min)

$$\text{R} = \frac{\text{V} \times \text{D}}{\text{T}}$$

$$= \frac{60 \times 15}{60}$$

$$= 15 \text{ drops/min, answer}$$

Example 3:

In pediatric patients, heparin sodium is administered by intermittent IV infusion in a range of 60 to 80 units/kg of body weight every 4 hrs. For a 60-lb child, calculate the range, in mL, of a heparin sodium injection containing 5000 units/mL to be administered daily.

$$60 \text{ lb}/2.2 = 27.27 \text{ kg}$$

$$(60 - 80) \times 24/4 = (360 - 480)$$

$$(360 - 480) \times 27.27 \text{ kg} = (9817 - 13,090)$$

$$\frac{5000 \text{ units}}{9817 \text{ units}} = \frac{1 \text{ mL}}{\text{X mL}}$$

$$\text{X} = 1.96 \text{ mL}$$

$$\frac{5000 \text{ units}}{13,090 \text{ units}} = \frac{1 \text{ mL}}{\text{X mL}}$$

$$\text{X} = 2.62 \text{ mL}$$

Therefore the range = 1.96 to 2.62 mL, answer

PRACTICE PROBLEMS

1. A patient is to receive an IV drip of the following:

Sodium Heparin	15,000 units
Sodium Chloride Injection (0.45%)	1000 mL

   a. How many milliliters per hour must be administered to achieve a rate of 2000 units of sodium heparin per hour?
   b. If the IV set delivers 10 drops/mL, how many drops per minute should be administered?
2. A patient is to receive an IV drip of the following:

Sodium Heparin	5,000 units
Sodium Chloride Injection (0.45%)	100 mL

   a. How many milliliters per hour must be administered to achieve a rate of 1000 units of sodium heparin per hour?
   b. If the IV set delivers 15 drops/mL, how many drops per minute should be administered?
3. A patient is to receive an IV drip of the following:

Sodium Heparin	10,000 units
Sodium Chloride Injection (0.45%)	200 mL

   a. How many milliliters per hour must be administered to achieve a rate of 200 units of sodium heparin per hour?
   b. If the IV set delivers 100 drops/mL, how many drops per minute should be administered?

4. A patient is to receive an IV drip of the following:

Sodium Heparin	7,000 units
Sodium Chloride Injection	700 mL

   a. How many milliliters per hour must be administered to achieve a rate of 1000 units of sodium heparin per hour?
   b. If the IV set delivers 10 drops/mL, how many drops per minute should be administered?

5. A patient is to receive an IV drip of the following:

Sodium Heparin	50,000 units
Sodium Chloride Injection (0.45%)	1000 mL

   a. How many milliliters per hour must be administered to achieve a rate of 2000 units of sodium heparin per hour?
   b. If the IV set delivers 10 drops/mL, how many drops per minute should be administered?

6. A patient is to receive an IV drip of the following:

Heparin	4000 units
Sodium Chloride Injection (0.45%)	500 mL

   a. How many milliliters per hour must be administered to achieve a rate of 100 units of sodium heparin per hour?
   b. If the IV set delivers 20 drops/mL, how many drops per minute should be administered?

7. A patient is to receive an IV drip of the following:

Sodium Heparin	8000 units
Sodium Chloride Injection (0.45%)	100 mL

   a. How many milliliters per hour must be administered to achieve a rate of 4,000 units of sodium heparin per hour?
   b. If the IV set delivers 50 drops/mL, how many drops per minute should be administered?

8. A patient is to receive an IV drip of the following:

Sodium Heparin	6000 units
Sodium Chloride Injection (0.45%)	500 mL

   a. How many milliliters per hour must be administered to achieve a rate of 1000 units of sodium heparin per hour?
   b. If the IV set delivers 40 drops/mL, how many drops per minute should be administered?

9. A patient is to receive an IV drip of the following:

Sodium Heparin	9000 units
Sodium Chloride Injection (0.45%)	1000 mL

a. How many milliliters per hour must be administered to achieve a rate of 4500 units of sodium heparin per hour?
b. If the IV set delivers 10 drops/mL, how many drops per minute should be administered?

10. A patient is to receive an IV drip of the following:

Sodium Heparin	80,000 units
Sodium Chloride Injection (0.45%)	1000 mL

a. How many milliliters per hour must be administered to achieve a rate of 1000 units of sodium heparin per hour?
b. If the IV set delivers 50 drops/mL, how many drops per minute should be administered?

11. A heparin dose of 250 units/kg of body weight has been recommended for a patient undergoing surgery. How many mL of an injection containing 5000 heparin units/mL should be administered to a 120-lb patient?
12. A heparin dose of 120 units/lb of body weight has been recommended for a patient undergoing surgery. How many mL of an injection containing 4000 heparin units/mL should be administered to a 250-lb patient?
13. A patient receives 50 mL every hr. If 10 units are in each mL, how many units does the patient receive in 24 hr?
14. A heparin dose of 150 units/kg of body weight has been recommended for a patient undergoing surgery. How many mL of an injection containing 6000 heparin units/mL should be administered to a 100-lb patient?
15. A heparin dose of 100 units/kg of body weight has been recommended for a patient undergoing surgery. How many mL of an injection containing 5000 heparin units/mL should be administered to a 200-lb patient?
16. A heparin dose of 200 units/lb of body weight has been recommended for a patient undergoing surgery. How many mL of an injection containing 3000 heparin units/mL should be administered to a 220-lb patient?
17. A heparin dose of 160 units/kg of body weight has been recommended for a patient undergoing surgery. How many mL of an injection containing 1000 heparin units/mL should be administered to a 60-kg patient?
18. A heparin dose of 150 units/lb of body weight has been recommended for a patient undergoing surgery. How many mL of an injection containing 5000 heparin units/mL should be administered to a 50-kg patient?
19. A heparin dose of 50 mL/kg of body weight has been recommended for a patient undergoing surgery. How many units of an injection containing 500 heparin units/mL should be administered to a 220-lb patient?
20. A heparin dose of 100 units/lb of body weight has been recommended for a patient undergoing surgery. How many mL of an injection containing 2000 heparin units/mL should be administered to a 70-kg patient?
21. For children, heparin sodium is administered by intermittent IV infusion in a range of 60 to 80 units/kg of body weight every 4 hrs. For a 57-lb child, calculate the range, in mL, of a heparin sodium injection containing 5000 units/mL to be administered daily.

22. For children, heparin sodium is administered by intermittent IV infusion in a range of 70 to 90 units/kg of body weight every 4 hrs. For a 50-lb child, calculate the range, in mL, of a heparin sodium injection containing 5000 units/mL to be administered daily.
23. For children, heparin sodium is administered by intermittent IV infusion in a range of 65 to 85 units/kg of body weight every 4 hrs. For a 58-lb child, calculate the range, in mL, of a heparin sodium injection containing 5000 units/mL to be administered daily.
24. For children, heparin sodium is administered by intermittent IV infusion in a range of 70 to 90 units/kg of body weight every 4 hrs. For a 60-lb child, calculate the range, in mL, of a heparin sodium injection containing 8000 units/mL to be administered daily.
25. For children, heparin sodium is administered by intermittent IV infusion in a range of 65 to 80 units/kg of body weight every 4 hrs. For a 70-lb child, calculate the range, in mL, of a heparin sodium injection containing 5000 units/mL to be administered daily.
26. For children, heparin sodium is administered by intermittent IV infusion in a range of 70 to 85 units/kg of body weight every 6 hrs. For a 68-lb child, calculate the range, in mL, of a heparin sodium injection containing 1000 units/mL to be administered daily.
27. For children, heparin sodium is administered by intermittent IV infusion in a range of 70 to 80 units/kg of body weight every 4 hrs. For a 100-lb child, calculate the range, in mL, of a heparin sodium injection containing 2000 units/mL to be administered daily.
28. For children, heparin sodium is administered by intermittent IV infusion in a range of 80 to 100 units/kg of body weight every 4 hrs. For a 100-lb child, calculate the range, in mL, of a heparin sodium injection containing 1000 units/mL to be administered daily.
29. For children, heparin sodium is administered by intermittent IV infusion in a range of 100 to 120 units/kg of body weight every 4 hrs. For a 60-lb child, calculate the range, in mL, of a heparin sodium injection containing 4000 units/mL to be administered daily.
30. Calculate the number of units per milliliter if a 4 mL vial of heparin containing 10,000 units/mL is injected into 1000 mL of normal saline solution.
31. Calculate the number of units per milliliter if an 8 mL vial of heparin containing 8,000 units/mL is injected into 1000 mL of normal saline solution.
32. Calculate the number of units per milliliter if a 5 mL vial of heparin containing 8,000 units/mL is injected into 5000 mL of normal saline solution.
33. Calculate the number of units per milliliter if a 2 mL vial of heparin containing 20,000 units/mL is injected into 500 mL of normal saline solution.

34. Calculate the number of units per milliliter if a 20 mL vial of heparin containing 60,000 units/mL is injected into 500 mL of normal saline solution.
35. Calculate the number of units per milliliter if a 3 mL vial of heparin containing 200,000 units/mL is injected into 1000 mL of normal saline solution.
36. Calculate the number of units per milliliter if a 25 mL vial of heparin containing 60,000 units/mL is injected into 500 mL of normal saline solution.
37. Calculate the number of units per milliliter if a 9 mL vial of heparin containing 20,000 units/mL is injected into 1000 mL of normal saline solution.
38. Calculate the number of units per milliliter if a 10 mL vial of heparin containing 30,000 units/mL is injected into 250 mL of normal saline solution.
39. Calculate the number of units per milliliter if an 8 mL vial of heparin containing 25,000 units/mL is injected into 500 mL of normal saline solution.
40. Calculate the number of units per milliliter if a 6 mL vial of heparin containing 100,000 units/mL is injected into 500 mL of normal saline solution.
41. A patient receives 30 mL of heparin every hour. If there are 40 units in each mL, how many units does the patient receive in 24 hrs?
42. A patient receives 90 mL of heparin every 2 hours. If there are 80 units in each mL, how many units does the patient receive in 24 hrs?
43. A patient receives 8 mL of heparin every 6 hours. If there are 10 units in each mL, how many units does the patient receive in 24 hrs?
44. A patient receives 10 mL of heparin every 12 hours. If there are 100 units in each mL, how many units does the patient receive in 24 hrs?
45. A patient receives 80 mL of heparin every 6 hours. If there are 900 units in each mL, how many units does the patient receive in 24 hrs?
46. A patient receives 10 mL of heparin every 3 hours. If there are 90 units in each mL, how many units does the patient receive in 24 hrs?
47. A patient receives 8 mL of heparin every 6 hours. If there are 200 units in each mL, how many units does the patient receive in 2 days?
48. A patient receives 50 mL of heparin every hour. If there are 100 units in each mL, how many units does the patient receive in 3 days?
49. A patient receives 80 mL of heparin every 2 hours. If there are 800 units in each mL, how many units does the patient receive in 2 days?
50. A patient receives 50 mL of heparin every 6 hours. If there are 25 units in each mL, how many units does the patient receive in 2 days?

ANSWERS

Insulin

1. b
2. a
3. d
4. c
5. b
6. b
7. c
8. b
9. b
10. d
11. d
12. d
13. c
14. d
15. c
16. b
17. 1.72 mL/day
18. 109.1 or 109 units/day
19. 66.53 or 66.5 units/day
20. 1.0 mL/day
21. 209 units/day
22. 8.11, or 8 mL/day
23. 12 units of U-500 Iletin I insulin /day
24. 48 units of U-500 Iletin I insulin /day
25. 30 mL of U-100 mixtard insulin/day
26. 60 units of U-100 protamine zinc insulin /day
27. 1500 mL of U-100 mixtard insulin/day
28. 75 units of U-100 humulin insulin
29. 200 units of humulin insulin
30. 71.5 or 72 units of protamine zinc insulin
31. 102.3 or 102 units of U-100 velosulin insulin
32. 5.05 or 5.1 mL/day of protamine zinc insulin
33. 40 U of mixtard insulin and 20 U of isophane insulin
34. 1.25 mL of isophane insulin and 50 units of protamine zinc
35. 60 units of U-40 lent insulin and 70 units of velosulin human insulin
36. 0.15 mL of U-100 protamine zinc insulin and 0.6 mL of U-40 isophane insulin
37. 0.625 mL of U-40 regular Iletin I and 0.01 mL of U-500 concentrated Iletin II
38. 0.75 mL of U-40 NPH Iletin and 0.8 mL of U-100 isulatard NPH
39. 30 units of U-40 isophane insulin

40. 0.2 mL of U-100 human insulin and 0.1 mL of U-100 protamine zinc insulin
41. 1×10^5 of U-100 humulin insulin and, 6×10^5 of U-400 mixtard for the entire month
42. 200 units
43. 1.6 mL of insulin
44. 84 units of U-40 isophane insulin and 292 units of U-100 mixtard insulin
45. 30 units of U-100 ultralent insulin and 20 units of U-100 humulin insulin
46. 4.13 mL insulin
47. 43 units of U-40 NPH Iletin I and, 67 units of U-100 humulin insulin
48. 56 units of U-40 isophane, and 60 units of U-100 mixtard insulin
49. 1000 vials of each
50. 400 vials

Heparin

1. 133.3 mL and 22 drops
2. 20 mL/hr and 5 drops/min
3. 4 mL/hr and 6.67 drops/min
4. 100 mL/hr and 18 drops/min
5. 40 mL/hr and 6.67 drops/min
6. 12.5 mL/hr and 4.16 drops/min
7. 50 mL/hr and 41.6 drops/min
8. 83.33 mL/hr and 55.55 drops/min
9. 500 mL/hr and 83.3 drops/min
10. 12.5 mL/hr and 10.4 drops/min
11. 2.73 mL
12. 7.5 mL
13. 12000 units
14. 1.14 mL
15. 1.82 mL
16. 14.66 mL
17. 9.6 mL
18. 3.3 mL
19. 2500000 units
20. 7.7 mL
21. 1.63 to 2.48 mL
22. 1.9 to 2.45 mL
23. 2.05 to 2.68 mL
24. 1.4 to 1.83 mL
25. 2.84 3.05 mL
26. 8.6 to 10.6 mL
27. 9.5 to 10.8 mL
28. 21.7 to 27.2 mL
29. 4.08 to 4.8 mL
30. 40 units/mL
31. 64 units/mL
32. 8 units/mL
33. 80 units/mL
34. 240 units/mL
35. 600 units/mL
36. 3,000 units/mL
37. 180 units/mL
38. 1,200 units/mL
39. 400 units/mL
40. 1,200 units/mL
41. 2,880 units
42. 86,400 units
43. 320 units
44. 2,000 units
45. 288,000 units
46. 7,200 units
47. 12,800 units
48. 360,000 units
49. 1,536,000 units
50. 10,000 units

APPENDIX A

Working with Temperature Conversions

The intensity of heat, or temperature, is measured in Celsius (centigrade) or Fahrenheit scales, and expressed in degrees (°). The instrument that measures the temperature is called thermometer. Most thermometers in the U.S. use the Fahrenheit scale.

The Fahrenheit (F) scale establishes the freezing point of pure water at 32°F and the boiling point at 212°F. The Celsius scale establishes freezing at 0°C and boiling at 100°C. The difference between boiling and freezing points in the Fahrenheit scale is 180 and in Celsius is 100. Each Celsius degree is equal to 180/100 or 1.8°F. By rounding the numbers one can express the same as "every 5 degrees measured in the Celsius scale is equal to 9 degrees as measured by the Fahrenheit scale."

CONVERSION FROM °F TO °C

To convert the temperature from Fahrenheit scale to Celsius scale, the following expression may be used:

$$°C = \frac{°F - 32}{1.8}$$

Example 1:

Convert 72°F to °C.

$$°C = \frac{°F - 32}{1.8}$$

$$°C = \frac{72 - 32}{1.8}$$

$$°C = 22.22$$

Example 2:

Convert 92°F to °C.

$$°C = \frac{92 - 32}{1.8}$$

$$°C = 33.33$$

Example 3:

Convert 20°F to °C.

$$°C = \frac{°F - 32}{1.8}$$

$$°C = \frac{20 - 32}{1.8}$$

$$°C = -6.67$$

CONVERSION FROM °C TO °F

To convert the temperature from Celsius scale to Fahrenheit scale, the following expression may be used:

$$°F = (1.8 \times °C) + 32$$

Example 1:

Convert 0°C to °F.

$$°F = (1.8 \times °C) + 32$$

$$°F = 32$$

Example 2:

Convert 45°C to °F.

$$°F = (1.8 \times °C) + 32$$

$$°F = 113$$

Example 3:

Convert 75°C to °F.

$$°F = (1.8 \times °C) + 32$$

$$°F = 167$$

PRACTICE PROBLEMS

Conversion from °F to °C

1. Convert the normal body temperature of 98.6°F to °C.
2. The temperature of the oil was 162°F. What would be the temperature in °C?
3. The temperature on an island was –58°F. What would be the temperature in °C?
4. The binding study is normally done at 8°F. Convert it to °C.
5. The temperature of liquid nitrogen is –180°F. Convert this to °C.
6. It was found that an analgesic drug could be recrystallized at a temperature of –67°F. What is the temperature of recrystallization in °C?
7. Insulin injection should be stored in the refrigerator at 39.2°F. Convert this temperature to °C.
8. A novel drug remains stable for 5 years if stored at 28°F. Express this temperature in °C.
9. The freeze-drying of a protein solution can be done at –150°F. What is this temperature in °C?
10. A liquid is known to solidify at 10°F. What is this temperature in °C?
11. Convert –90°F to °C.
12. The summer temperature in the Texas Panhandle is usually 80°F. What is this temperature in °C?
13. The permeability of ketoconazole through rat intestine was estimated at 100°F. What is this temperature in °C?
14. Nitroglycerine tablets should be stored at 77°F. Express this storage condition in °C.
15. The degradation of aspirin increases 1.5 times if temperature is raised from 85°F to 95°F. Express this range in °C.

Conversion from °C to °F

16. Convert 26°C to °F.
17. Convert –35°C to °F.
18. Convert 20°C to °F.
19. The freezing point of pure water is 0°C. Convert this to °F.
20. The boiling point of pure water is 100°C. Convert this to °F.
21. Certain stability studies are done at 60°C. Convert this temperature to °F.
22. Calamine lotion stored at 40°C was found to be degraded. What is this temperature in °F?
23. Paracetamol tablets if stored below 30°C remain stable for 3 years. What is this temperature in °F?
24. Cocoa butter melts at body temperature of 37°C. What is this temperature in °F?
25. Furosemide degrades at temperatures above 58°C. What is this temperature in °F?
26. Protamine sulfate tablets should be stored at 5°C. What is this temperature in °F?

27. Aluminum hydroxide suspension separates at 50°C. Express this temperature in °F.
28. Calcitonin solution remains stable at 4°C for 10 days. Express this temperature in °F.
29. Coenzyme Q10 tablets are most stable at a temperature of 22°C. What is this temperature in °F?
30. The cimetidine degradation rate doubles if temperature is increased from 20 to 30°C. Express these temperatures in °F.

ANSWERS

Conversion from °F to °C

1. 37
2. 72.2
3. –50
4. –13.3
5. –117.8
6. –55
7. 4
8. –2.2
9. –101
10. –12.2
11. –67.8
12. 26.7
13. 37.8
14. 25
15. 29.4 and 35

Conversion from °C to °F

16. 78.8
17. –31
18. 68
19. 32
20. 212
21. 140
22. 104
23. 86
24. 98.6
25. 136.4
26. 41
27. 122
28. 39.2
29. 71.6
30. 35.6, 37.4

Appendix B
Working with Capsule Dosage Forms

Pharmacists and technicians play an important role in filling hard gelatin capsules. Many times, a combination of drugs is compounded in capsules. For the compounding of capsules, powdered ingredients are accurately weighed, mixed by the geometric dilution method, and filled in appropriately sized capsules. Sometimes if the powdered ingredients are not readily available, they can be obtained by crushing the available tablets. Lactose or other diluents may be needed to make up the volume of powder to fill in the capsules.

Hard gelatin capsules are available in a range of sizes such as 00, 0, 1, 2, 3, 4, and 5, which represent a gradual decrease in size from 00 to 5. The largest capsule size, represented as 000, is rarely used. The hard gelatin capsules consist of a cylindrical body and a cap. The cap is slightly larger and broader but shorter, and the body is narrower and longer. The medication is filled in the body, following which the cap is fitted over it. Select the capsules of smallest size that will hold the quantity of powdered material. To figure the size of the capsule needed, accurately weighed powdered material is usually filled in one or two capsules as a trial. If the size is appropriate, then the rest of the material is filled in capsules of the same size. When the bulk density of powders is 0.6 g/cc, the size of the capsule can be approximated by the rule of sixes. According to this rule, capsule sizes, 0, 1, 2, 3, 4, and 5 can hold 6–7, 5, 4, 3, 2, and ½–1 grains of the powders, respectively. Each grain is approximately equivalent to 65 mg.

COMPOUNDING TIPS AND CALCULATIONS FOR FILLING CAPSULES

In order to fill capsules as a dosage form, the following steps may be helpful.

Step 1. Determine whether the prescription is based upon one unit or upon a bulk formula to be subdivided into individual units. *Subscription* of the prescriptions is very important for this determination. For example, *M et Div* suggests that the prescription is written for some bulk formula which is to be subdivided into individual capsules. On the other hand, *D.T.D.* in the *subscription* suggests that the formula is given for one capsule, and depending upon the number of capsules needed in the prescription, the formula quantities should be multiplied.

Step 2. Determine the weight of each ingredient in the formula, weigh accurately, and mix the ingredients by the geometric mixing technique. If the ingredients have to be obtained from commercial tablets, determine the appropriate number of tablets needed, crush them, and weigh out the material. Then proceed as with powders.

Step 3. Determine the capsule size by using the rule of sixes. If the amount of total powder is less than the desired amount in the capsule, add suitable amount of a diluent, preferably lactose, to make up the volume. Fill one or two capsules to confirm the size. If the size is correct, "punch" out the remaining capsules after forming a 'cake" on a powder paper. An ointment tile may also be used.

Step 4. Wipe all the capsules from outside with a clean tissue paper, and dispense the capsules in an appropriate container after affixing the label. Contents of the label and the need for any auxiliary label will depend upon the nature of the medication.

Example 1:

Show the calculations to determine the number of HCTZ 50 mg and triamterene 50 mg tablets to fill the prescription.

Henry Huxtable, M.D.
61-40 Flushing Avenue
Amarillo, TX 79106
Phone No. 555-1234

Name : Sonya Burns **Age**: 36
Address: 96 Havana Blvd., TX 79106 **Date**: 3/18/03

℞

Hydrochlorothiazide	20 mg
Triamterene	40 mg
Lactose q.s.	

M. ft caps. DTD # 10

Sig: i cap bid, UD

REFILL 1 x

DAW ______

HHuxtable
DEA # AD 7973142

Tablets available: HCTZ 50 mg and Triamterene 50 mg

Procedure:

Step 1: The prescription is based upon one capsule, and Dr. Huxtable wants 10 such capsules for his patient, Ms. Burns.

Step 2: 20 mg × 10 = 200 mg of hydrochlorthiazide and 40 mg × 10 = 400 mg of triamterene are needed for the ten capsules that are required for the prescription. Since bulk powders are not provided, the available tablets of hydrochlorthiazide and triamterene should be used. The number of tablets to be crushed is determined by using the following proportion:

$$\frac{50 \text{ mg of HCTZ}}{1 \text{ tablet}} = \frac{200 \text{ mg of HCTZ}}{\text{X tablets}}$$

$$\text{X} = 4 \text{ tablets of HCTZ}$$

$$\frac{50 \text{ mg of triamterene}}{1 \text{ tablet}} = \frac{400 \text{ mg of triamterene}}{\text{X tablets}}$$

$$\text{X} = 8 \text{ tablets of triamterene}$$

Example 2:

Show the detailed method of compounding the following prescription along with all the calculations.

Henry Huxtable, M.D.
61-40 Flushing Avenue
Amarillo, TX 79106
Phone No. 555-1234

Name : Frank Bruno **Age**: 32
Address: 142 Garden Street, TX-79121 **Date**: 3/16/03

℞

Ephedrine Sulfate	0.30 g
Phenobarbital	0.18 g
Lactose qs	

Ft. caps. M et Div. #12

Sig: i cap bid

REFILL None

DAW ________

HHuxtable
DEA # AD 7973142

Procedure:

Step 1: The prescription is based upon 12 capsules, i.e., the ingredient quantities given (Ephedrine sulfate 0.3 g and Phenobarbital 0.018 g) are for 12 capsules.

Step 2: Weigh 300 milligrams of ephedrine sulfate and 180 mg of phenobarbital and mix thoroughly. The total quantity of the mixture of these two powders is 480 mg. The amount of ephedrine sulfate needed for one capsule is 25 mg (300 mg of powder/12 capsules) and that of phenobarbital is 15 mg (180 mg of powder/12 capsules). The total amount of powdered drugs in each capsule is 40 mg.

Step 3: By the *rule of sixes*, capsule size #2 can hold a total powder quantity of about 2 grains or130 mg. Considering this amount, the total amount of powder for 12 capsules of size #2 is 1560 mg. The amount of lactose that should be added for 12 capsules is 1080 mg (calculated as 1560 mg – 480 mg = 1080 mg). Therefore, weigh 1080 mg of lactose and add to the drug mixture by geometric dilution. As a confirmation of the size, fill one or two capsules of size #2 with 130 mg of the mixture and determine the appropriateness. If the capsule size is correct, punch out the remaining capsules after forming a cake on a powder paper or an ointment tile.

Step 4: Wipe all the capsules from outside with a clean and dry tissue, and submit in an appropriate container after affixing the following label:

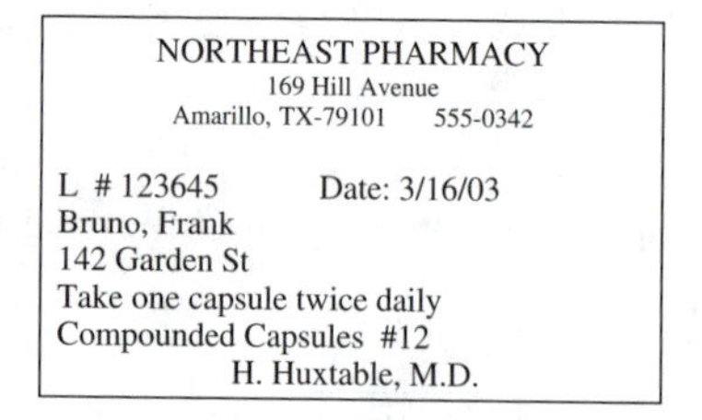

NORTHEAST PHARMACY
169 Hill Avenue
Amarillo, TX-79101 555-0342

L # 123645 Date: 3/16/03
Bruno, Frank
142 Garden St
Take one capsule twice daily
Compounded Capsules #12
H. Huxtable, M.D.

PRACTICE PROBLEMS

The following ten prescriptions are for capsules which are to be prepared either from bulk chemicals or tablets, the information about which will be provided following each prescription. For all the prescriptions, check if the *subscription* is correct and provide all the steps that you will follow to fill the prescription. Make sure that you show all the calculations involved, the capsule size selected, and the label for final container.

Patrick King, M.D.
61-40 Flushing Avenue
Amarillo, TX-79106
Phone No. 555-1234

Name: Piper Doe **Age**: 32
Address: 96 Main St., TX-79106 **Date**: 3/9/03

℞
Aldomet 1.2 g
Hydralazine 0.1 g
Lactose qs 3.25 g

Ft. caps. # 10

Sig: i cap qid

REFILL None

DAW ______

PKing
Lic # 333444

Available tablets: Methyldopa 500 mg weighing one gram each, and Hydralazine tablets 50 mg weighing 200 mg each.

2.

Patrick King, M.D.
13 Main St.
Amarillo, TX 79101
Phone No. 555-1234

Name : Magic Jordan **Age**: 32
Address: 96 Sheldon St, TX-79106 **Date**: 3/9/03

℞
Hydralazine HCl 10 mg
HCTZ 20 mg
Lactose qs

Ft. caps. # xiv

Sig: i 8 A.M., and 4 P.M.

REFILL None

DAW ________

PKing
Lic # 333444

Available tablets: Hydralazine HCl 50 mg weighing 200 mg each, and HCTZ 20 mg tablets weighing 160 mg each.

3.

Patrick King, M.D.
13 Main Street
Amarillo, TX 79106
Phone No. 555-1234

Name : Michael Johnson **Age**: 32
Address: 21 Progress Dr, TX 79106 **Date**: 3/9/03

℞
CPM 5 mg
Pseudoephedrine HCl 40 mg
ASA 300 mg
Lactose qs ad

Ft. caps. DTD # 12

Sig: i cap q6h

REFILL None

DAW ________

PKing
Lic # 333444

Available: Bulk powders of all the ingredients.

4.

Patrick King, M.D.
13 Main Street
Amarillo, TX 79106
Phone No. 555-1234

Name : Tim Johnson **Age**: 32
Address: 13 Victory Dr., TX 79106 **Date**: 3/9/03

℞

Dimenhydrinate	
Pantothenic acid aa	30 mg
Thiamine HCl	10 mg
Calcium carbonate	100 mg

M. Ft. cap DTD #12
Sig: i cap qid for nausea

REFILL None

PKing
Lic # 333444

Available: Bulk powder of dimenhydrinate and pantothenic acid, 25 mg tablets of thiamine HCl weighing 200 mg each, and 500 mg tablets of calcium carbonate weighing one gram each.

5.

Patrick King, M.D.
13 Main Street
Amarillo, TX 79106
Phone No. 555-1234

Name : Gunn Hermann **Age**: 34
Address: 13 Coulter St, TX 79106 **Date**: 3/9/03

℞

ASA	175 mg
Ephedrine sulfate	20 mg
CPM	2 mg

Ft. caps. D.T.D. # 12

Sig: i cap q6h, prn

REFILL None

PKing
Lic # 333444

Available: 325 mg aspirin tablets weighing 0.7 g each, 60 mg ephedrine sulfate weighing 200 mg each, and 4 mg cpm weighing 150 mg each.

6.

Patrick King, M.D.
13 Main Street
Amarillo, TX 79106
Phone No. 555-1234

Name : Vicky Johnson **Age**: 23
Address: 13 Bell St. TX 79106 **Date**: 3/9/03

℞

Diphenhydramine HCl	20 mg
Prednisone	2. 5 mg
Lactose qs ad	300 mg

Sig: i cap q8h

M.Ft Cap. DTD XV

REFILL None

DAW

PKing
Lic # 333444

Available: 50 mg Benadryl capsules weighing 200 mg, and 4 mg prednisone tablets weighing 180 mg each.

7.

Patrick King, M.D.
13 Main Street
Amarillo, TX 79106
Phone No. 555-1234

Name : Latina Davis **Age**: 21
Address: 21 Bell St., TX 79106 **Date**: 3/9/03

℞

Simethicone	0.02 g
Phenobarb.	0.075 g
Magnesium carbonate	0.05 g

M. Ft caps D.T.D. # 12
Sig: ii caps tid & HS

REFILL None

DAW

PKing
Lic # 333444

Available: 20 mg simethicone tablets weighing 150 mg each, phenobarbital powder, and 500 mg magnesium carbonate tablets weighing one gram each.

8.

Patrick King, M.D.
13 Main Street
Amarillo, TX 79106
Phone No. 555-1234

Name : Hill Grant **Age**: 24
Address: 2101 WestCliff, TX-79101 **Date**: 3/9/03

℞
Warfarin sodium 1.5 mg
Lactose qs ad 300 mg

M.Ft. Cap D.T.D. # xii

Sig: i qAM

REFILL None

DAW

PKing
Lic # 333444

Tablets available: 5 mg warfarin sodium tablets weighing 150 mg each.

9.

Patrick King, M.D.
13 Main Street
Amarillo, TX 79106
Phone No. 555-1234

Name : Karl Mailman **Age**: 5 Yr
Address: 13 Bell St., TX 79106 **Date**: 3/9/03
Weight = 44 lbs

℞
Sulfasalazine 40 mg/kg/24 hours
Prednisone 1 mg/cap
Lactose qs

Ft. caps. DTD # 15

Sig: Contents of i capsule in applesauce q6h

DAW

PKing
Lic # 333444

Bulk powders for all the ingredients are available.

10.

Patrick King, M.D.
13 Main Street
Amarillo, TX 79106
Phone No. 555-1234

Name : Dennis Menace **Age**: 32
Address: 2101 Hill Dr., TX 79106 **Date**: 3/9/03

℞

CPM	2 mg
APAP	350 mg
Pseudoephed sulfate	30 mg
Lactose qs	

Ft. caps. DTD # xv

Sig: ii caps, prn for sinus headache

REFILL None

DAW

PKing
Lic # 333444

Bulk powders are available for all the ingredients.

Appendix C

Dealing with Pediatric Dosages

The remarkable differences between adults and children necessitate a special consideration in dealing with the pediatric doses and dosage regimens. These differences arise from many factors including changes in pharmacokinetic parameters, age, body weight and composition, surface area, and genetic predisposition. Following are some calculations based on body weight, height, surface area, and age.

BASED ON BODY WEIGHT

Clark's rule. This can be used to estimate the appropriate pediatric dose from the adult dose based on body weight in pounds.

$$\text{Child dose} = \left((\text{child's weight in pounds})/150\right) \times (\text{adult dose})$$

where 150 is the average adult weight in pounds.

BASED ON HEIGHT

One way of dosing a child is to give the proportion of the adult dose based on child's height relative to the average adult height.

$$\text{Pediatric dose} = (\text{child's height in centimeters}/174) \times (\text{adult dose})$$

where 174 is the average adult height in centimeters (68.5 inches).

BASED ON BODY SURFACE AREA (BSA)

One way of dosing a child is to give the proportion of the adult dose based on the child's body surface area (BSA) relative to that seen with the average adult.

$$\text{Pediatric dose} = \left((\text{child's BSa in square meters})/1.73\right) \times (\text{adult dose})$$

where 1.73 is the average adult BSA in square meters.

BASED ON AGE

This method (a.k.a. *Webster's Rule*) allows an estimation of the appropriate pediatric dose from the adult dose based on the child's age in years.

$$Child\ dose = \frac{Age\ in\ years + 1}{Age\ in\ years + 7} \times adult\ dose$$

OTHER FORMULAS USED

Young's Rule

$$Child\ dose = \frac{Age\ in\ years}{Age + 12} \times Adult\ dose$$

Note: Young's Rule is preferably used for children between 1 to 12 years of age.

Drilling's Rule

$$Child\ dose = \frac{Age\ in\ years \times adult\ dose}{12}$$

Fried's Rule

$$Child\ dose = \frac{Age\ in\ months \times adult\ dose}{150}$$

Note: Fried's Rule is preferably used for infants up to 2 years of age.

PRACTICE PROBLEMS

1. The adult dose of drug A is 9 gr/day. Using Young's Rule, calculate the dose for a 6-year-old child.
2. The adult dose of a drug B is 5 gr. Using Young's Rule, calculate the dose for a 4 year-old child.
3. Using Clark's Rule, calculate the dose for a 30-lb child if the average adult dose is 500 mg/day.
4. Using Clark's Rule, calculate the dose for a 20-kg child if the average adult dose is 50 mg/day.
5. Using Clark's Rule, calculate the dose for a 50-lb child if the average adult dose is 0.9 g/day.
6. Using Fried's Rule, calculate the dose of medication A for a 15-month-old infant, if the adult dose is 100 mg.

7. Using the most appropriate rule, calculate the dose of medication A for a 10-month-old infant, if the adult dose is 30 mg.
8. The daily adult dose of Velosef capsule is up to 3 g/day. Using Young's Rule, calculate the dose for a 4-year-old child.
9. What is the dose for a 25-lb child, if the adult dose of a medication is 5 mg?
10. If the adult dose of a new analgesic drug is 150 mg, what is the dose for a child that has a body surface area of 0.7 m^2, given the average adult surface is 1.73 m^2?
11. If the adult dose of a drug B is 50 mg, what is the dose for a child that has a body surface area of 0.4 m^2?

ANSWERS

1. 3 gr
2. 1.25 gr
3. 100 mg
4. 14.67 mg
5. 0.3 g or 300 mg
6. 10 mg
7. Use Fried's Rule, 2 mg
8. 0.75 g/day
9. Use Clark's Rule, 0.83 mg
10. 60.7 mg
11. 11.56 mg

APPENDIX D

Pharmacy Business Math

The pharmacy personnel deal with a variety of business calculations involving markup, discount, depreciation, net profit, inventory control, salaries, overtime, overhead, and insurance. Pharmacy technicians should have a basic knowledge of numerical concepts and simple equations that are routinely encountered in their practice. Some examples illustrating pharmacy business calculations are presented below:

Example 1:

The purchase price of 100-count, 5-mg tablets of Clarinex is $232.60. If the dispensing cost is $55.20 and the profit goal is 25%, what should be the selling price for this product?

Note. The dispensing cost includes the costs of storing, handling, and other incidental expenses.

Purchase price = $232.60
Cost to dispense = $55.20
Overall cost = purchase price + cost to dispense
= $232.60 + $55.20
= $287.80
Net profit = overall cost × fraction of profit goal
= $287.80 × 0.25
= $71.95
Selling price = overall cost + net profit
= $287.80 + $71.95
= $359.75, answer

Example 2:

A 30-day supply of 20 mg tablets of Zocor sells for $164.90. If it costs only $137.50 to the pharmacy, calculate the markup and markup rate.

Purchase price = $137.50
Selling price = $164.90
Markup = selling price – purchase price
= 164.90 – 137.50
= $27.40

$$\begin{aligned}\text{Markup rate} &= (\text{markup} \div \text{purchase price}) \times 100\\ &= (27.40/137.50) \times 100\\ &= 20\%, \text{ answer}\end{aligned}$$

Example 3:

Corner Drug Store announces a 30% discount on a certain brand of cough syrup. If a bottle of this syrup is priced at $4.30, what should be the discounted price?

$$\begin{aligned}\text{Original price} &= \$4.30\\ \text{Discount} &= \text{original price} \times \text{discount rate}\\ &= 4.30 \times 0.30\\ &= \$1.29\\ \text{Discounted price} &= \text{original price} - \text{discount}\\ &= 4.40 - 1.29\\ &= \$3.11, \text{ answer}\end{aligned}$$

Example 4:

A neighborhood pharmacy store has an average inventory of $48,525 and has total annual purchases of $171,820. What is the turnover rate for this pharmacy?

$$\begin{aligned}\text{Cost of average inventory} &= \$48{,}525.00\\ \text{Total annual purchases} &= \$171{,}820.00\\ \text{Turnover rate} &= \text{total annual purchases} \div \text{cost of average inventory}\\ &= 171{,}820.00/48{,}525.00\\ &= 3.54 \text{ times, answer}\end{aligned}$$

Example 5:

A certain type of topical herbal skin care cream is priced at $12 but if this product is purchased within a week, a 40% discount is offered on the purchase price. What is the discounted price?

$$\begin{aligned}\text{Original purchase price} &= \$12.0\\ \text{Discount} &= \text{original purchase price} \times \text{discount rate}\\ &= 12.00 \times 0.40\\ &= \$4.80\\ \text{Discounted purchase price} &= \text{original purchase price} - \text{discount}\\ &= 12.00 - 4.80\\ &= \$7.20, \text{ answer}\end{aligned}$$

PRACTICE PROBLEMS

1. Doxycycline capsules cost $58 for a bottle that contains 50 tablets. If the store profit goal is 30%, what is the total selling price for this product?
2. Toprol XL 50 mg tablets costs a pharmacy $76. If the profit goal is 20%, what should be the selling price?
3. A certain type of allergy medication costs $45.80 for a month's supply. If the selling price is $52.70, what is the markup rate?
4. A 60-day supply of Zocor tablets sells for $320.60. If it costs only $236 to the pharmacy, what is the markup rate?
5. A three-month supply of vitamin supplements sells for $22. If it costs only $16.60 to the pharmacy, what is the markup?
6. Fincher's Pharmacy Store offers a 25% discount on a brand of cough syrup. If a bottle is priced at $3.60, what should be the discounted price?
7. Dawn Corner Store Pharmacy offers a 20% discount on a brand of cold medication. If a bottle of this cold medication is priced at $8.20, what should be the discounted price?
8. A type of topical anti-oxidant cream is priced at $5.60, but if this product is purchased within a week, a 20% discount is offered on the purchase price. What is the discounted price?
9. A high-volume retail pharmacy store has an average inventory of $258,400 and has total annual purchases of $1,085,280. What is the turnover rate for this pharmacy?
10. Down The Street Pharmacy has an average inventory of $38,650 and has total annual purchases of $115,950. What is the turnover rate for this pharmacy?

ANSWERS

1. $75.40
2. $91.20
3. 15%
4. 35.8%
5. $5.40
6. $2.70
7. $6.56
8. $4.48
9. 4.2
10. 3

Index

Note: Page numbers followed by a *t* refer to a table.

L

M

N

O

P

Q

R

S

T